Maximum Muscle
In Minimum Time

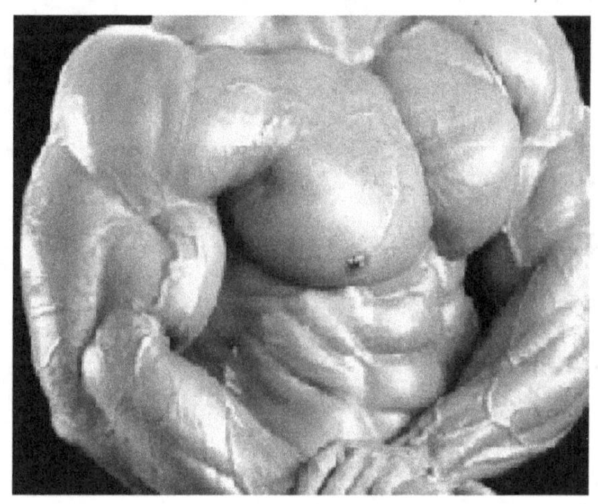

Complete Volume and HIT Training Programs

By David Groscup

IART/Med-Ex

HIT Trainer

Author of 8 Best-Selling Books On Bodybuilding Training

Table of Contents

There are many different forms of weight training beginning with the old time strongman kettle bell, which has become extremely popular because of its ability to develop explosive, functional strength using unique exercise movements. The dumbbell is one of the most versatile tools available because of its ability to provide the user with a longer range of motion than barbells and allowing one or two sides of the body to be exercised at one time.

Barbells are the most popular training tool and are used to effectively develop all parts of the physique using both compound and isolation movements. Machines appeared on the scene more recently than the others and are designed to pinpoint the resistance of an exercise on the target muscle using the proper range of motion.

All of these tools have their place in modern bodybuilding training and will be included in this book's training routines.

It's interesting to note that many of the old-school methods of training have made a comeback, and despite being around for awhile, have some merit and offer helpful insight into training techniques and unique exercises. Many famous bodybuilders of old designed a lot of these programs and were successful using them during their competitive careers and after they retired from active competition.

As scientific study of bodybuilding training methods were completed better ways of training were developed. These

include periodization, split routines and HIT to name a 4
few. One new technique that has become somewhat popular
in recent times is FS-T training. A moderate volume of
training is used with high rep "pump sets" to flush muscles
with large volumes of blood and nutrients. Stretching is used
to attempt to stretch the fascia, the membrane surrounding
the muscle to allow it to expand more easily.

The bodybuilding scene has practitioners that are "stuck" in
old-school methods, some of which have been proven to be
of limited benefit, while others are actively pursuing modern
methods to accelerate muscle growth faster than ever before.
The intelligent bodybuilder will attempt to rationally discern
what works best and discard the rest.

What This Book Will Do For You

Let me begin by telling you what this book won't do for you.
Since my other books explain in detail all of the advanced
techniques, or variables, available to you I will not explain
them in great detail in this volume. See my other book, DR
HIT's Effective High Intensity Variables for more
information.

In this book I will outline the best training routines to build
muscle fast using different approaches. If you are a volume
practitioner you will benefit. If you are like me, you will
derive great results from HIT, high intensity workouts. If you
fall somewhere in-between, you will use my workouts that
are designed around a modest set count. No matter which
training program you desire, you will find it here.

I will outline each workout clearly with complete 5
descriptions of all the exercises so you can implement them
in your training program immediately. Variations on training
principles will be presented , which allows great variety in
your program to prevent sticking points. Everything is
complementary to information contained in my other books
so readers will benefit from the information gleaned from
those.

Different viewpoints on training styles will be presented so
the reader can choose which method(s) to use in their
personal training to obtain the results they desire. Pros and
cons of all methods presented will be discussed and
variations and hybrids will be presented when appropriate.

The Origins of Bodybuilding

What are the origins of bodybuilding? How did bodybuilding
develop into such a popular pastime? Bodybuilding's
beginnings can be traced back to ancient Greek athletes who
used the lifting of weights to build strength, enabling them to
increase their skills in their chosen sport.

The most notable of such athletes was Olympic wrestling
champion Milo of Croton who reportedly would carry a calf
on his back every day until it became a bull, thus
demonstrating progressive resistance as a means of
developing strength.

Later, circus strongmen performed various feats of strength
during show performances. These feats of strength

included steel bar bending, lifting horses, horseshoe   6
bending, the tearing of license plates and decks of cards as
well as many other feats of strength. People admired these
men for their strength but didn't become impressed with the
looks of their physiques until Eugene Sandow came onto the
scene.

Born Friedrich Muller in 1867 in Prussia, Eugene Sandow
later became referred to as "The Father of Modern
Bodybuilding."

Sandow was incredibly strong, and while he wowed crowds
with his incredible strength and power, they were equally
impressed with the development of his muscular physique.

He initially traveled through Europe and later in the 1890's
America -- where he was billed as the "world's strongest
man". Sandow began using a posing routine to impress
crowds that came to see him perform.

Another influential figure in bodybuilding during the early
days was Bernarr Macfadden, who promoted bodybuilding
contests beginning in 1904 and produced a magazine,
Physical Culture Magazine, which was published for fifty
years.

He was largely responsible for the emergence of Charles
Atlas, who won the title of "World's Most Perfectly
Developed Man" in 1921. Atlas went on to market a training
course, "Dynamic Tension" which was designed to develop
young men's physiques by using a form of isometrics to build
strength and muscle.

He sold his course mainly through advertisements in   **7**
comic books -by showing a skinny man getting humiliated by
a big guy kicking sand in his face in front of bikini-clad
women. After training with Atlas's "Dynamic Tension," he
adds substantial muscle to his frame and impresses all of the
women on the beach by defeating the bully. It worked-Atlas
had quite a bit of success and sold many courses.

As time went on a new breed of bodybuilders such as Steve
Reeves came on the scene in the 40's and 50's. He not only
had good muscle mass but managed to build a symmetrical
physique by making sure his training was evenly balanced
between all muscle groups.

George Eiferman was another famous bodybuilder of this
era. He started lifting weights while in the Navy and
managed to add 40 lbs of muscle to his frame within a short
period of time. After leaving the Navy he joined a gym in
Philadelphia, PA and won the Mr. Philadelphia contest before
placing 5th in the Mr. America contest. One year later in 1948
he won the Mr. America title.

Eiferman continued to train and compete and won the Mr.
Universe in 1962. He helped train such luminaries as Steve
Reeves, Lou Ferrigno, and Arnold Schwarzenegger and
actors/actresses like Mae west, Debbie Reynolds, Liz Taylor
and Marilyn Monroe. He also helped train celebrities like
Rock Hudson, Sylvester Stallone, and even Elvis in the early
70's.

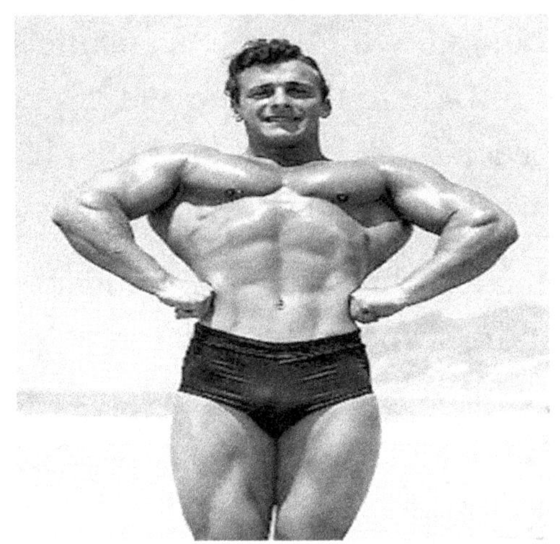

George Eiferman

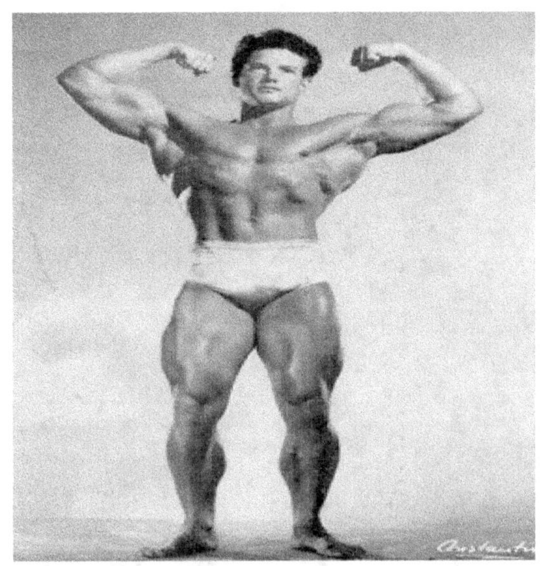

Steve Reeves

Other famous bodybuilders of the era are:

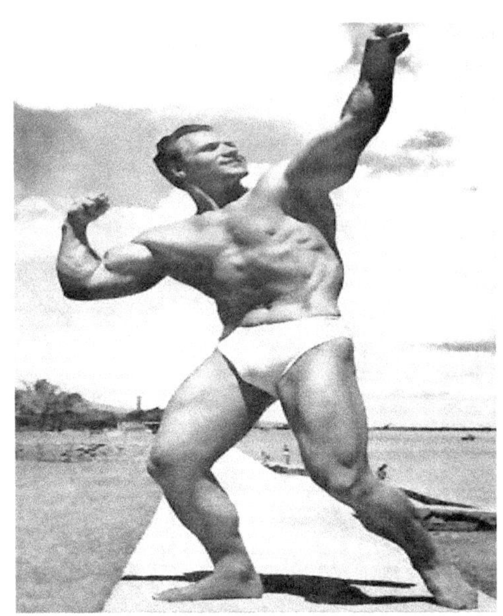

John Grimek of York Barbell Fame

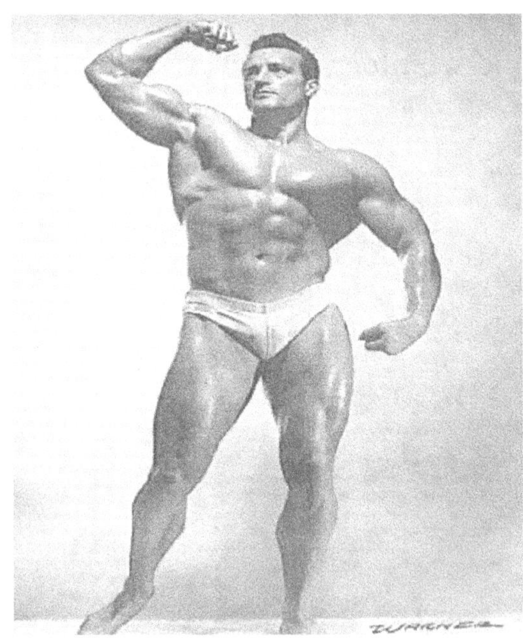

Clarence Ross

Explosion of Bodybuilding in the 70's and 80's   10

Many like myself, believe the golden era of bodybuilding was the 70's and early 80's. This is because of the rapidly growing popularity of bodybuilders of that time period. Names like Arnold Schwarzenegger and Lou Ferrigno helped make bodybuilding an up-and-coming sport, rumored to be possibly added to the Olympic games. Many young men aspired to look like their favorite bodybuilding champion and eagerly awaited next month's issue of Muscle Builder, Muscle Training Illustrated or Muscular Development.

The number of magazines grew and most of the top bodybuilding contests were televised on shows like 'Wide World of Sports'. Bodybuilding was featured in mainstream magazines and newspapers.

The fitness industry as a whole grew immensely during this time and gyms began popping up everywhere. Jack Lalane impressed the public with his feats of endurance and conditioning and hosted his own popular fitness/health television program. Golds gym in Venice Beach California became the mecca of bodybuilding, with all of the top champs training there at one time or another. The movie Pumping Iron became an immediate success, propelling Arnold Schwarzenegger to a household name.

Growth of Bodybuilding Steroids and Other Drugs and the Effect on the Bodybuilding Scene

In the late 70's the symmetrical physique began to gain in popularity, allowing Frank Zane, who was relatively small by the standard at the time, to win the coveted Mr. Olympia title three years in a row. That was short lived, however.

During this time bodybuilders became more massive due to hard training and the addition of steroid drugs, which were legal to use at the time. Although publicly denied, insiders knew what was happening with the growing steroid use. Eventually some bodybuilders "came clean" and admitted to the use of steroids and other drugs.

As things progressed additional pharmaceuticals were added such as HGH,human growth hormone and more recently Synthol, an oil-like substance that fills muscles and makes them larger. Things have gotten out of control, causing many of today's top professional bodybuilders to look like freaks to the general public. This has had the effect of making bodybuilding competitions limited to a cult-like following, which is unfortunate.

It's not unusual for today's bodybuilders to carry a lean body weight of 300 pounds at a height of 5'10", which is vastly heavier than bodybuilders as recent as the late 70's and 80's. In comparison, one famous bodybuilder of the 70's weighed 235 pounds at a height of 6'2" in contest shape. Many of today's bodybuilding stars look blocky with practically no symmetry.

The main reason for the increased body weight is the use of HGH, human growth hormone. This has greatly accelerated muscle growth over the use of anabolic steroids alone. Unfortunately it comes with its own set of dangerous side effects, especially in the high doses used today.

Natural Bodybuilding Contests

As a result of the drug use in bodybuilding and the desire of many bodybuilders to take part in a safe, healthy form of bodybuilding, natural bodybuilding contests were born. These events are tested by urinalysis alone so the effectiveness of the testing can be suspect. HGH, or human growth hormone is able to be detected by a blood test but doesn't show up in a urine test so this substance is used by some so-called natural bodybuilders to fool the governing agency and the testers.

This is unfortunate because I feel the natural contests are a step in the right direction. Since the majority of the competitors are natural-this is a great route to go for bodybuilders wanting to compete in a natural show.

Helpful Bodybuilding Supplements That promote Strength and Muscle Growth

There are an enormous amount of bodybuilding supplements on the market, with more coming virtually every day. Most use testimonials from top competitive bodybuilders to add credibility to the product to help sell it. Unfortunately, many of these products aren't used by these bodybuilders. This is a very deceitful practice used to sell high-priced supplements to amateur bodybuilders desperate to add muscle to their frames.

It is important to look at the research behind the claims being touted by the manufacturers and dealers behind these products before purchasing them to avoid wasting your 13 money.

One of the products that has conclusive proof of effectiveness is creatine monohydrate. It has been proven in many studies to be effective at increasing muscle strength and mass more than a placebo both in bodybuilding and non-bodybuilding populations. Creatine "pulls" water into the muscle adding to its size. This increases the protein synthesis in a muscle which increases muscle fiber growth.

Typically there is a loading phase, where a large dose is repeated daily for five days until the muscles are considered to be completely saturated. After that a daily dose, usually split into a morning and an evening dose, is continued indefinitely to maintain a steady increase of muscle size and strength.

Creatine has been shown to be beneficial to athletes that engage in bouts of high intensity anaerobic activities but hasn't demonstrated any benefit for ones that are involved in aerobic, or endurance activities.

Another helpful supplement is L-Glutamine, which is the amino acid found in the highest concentration in skeletal muscle tissue. In fact, over 61% of muscle is comprised of Glutamine. Glutamine consists of 19% nitrogen, making it the primary transporter of nitrogen into your muscle cells. It helps by limiting the breakdown of muscle tissue after a heavy bout of training, which enables the body to recover more quickly and build more muscle. Glutamine increases your body's ability to secrete Human Growth Hormone, which helps to burn body fat and support new muscle growth.

Boron supplementation has been promoted as an effective way to increase free testosterone. An athlete can have ample testosterone in their bloodstream but it is worthless if it is bound and unable to help develop muscle tissue. The most common binder is a protein called globulin. According to Quest Diagnostics, approximately 60 to 70 percent of testosterone in the blood binds to SHBG. Another 30 to 40 percent of circulating testosterone partners with albumin, which leaves only about 2 percent to circulate by itself in the free form.

The National Institutes of Health Pub Med website states that current research using placebo and Boron supplement groups found no benefit in increase of free testosterone from using Boron. This is unfortunate because Boron has been shown in other studies to reduce the incidence of prostate cancer in men who take Boron on a regular basis.

Zinc, on the other hand, was shown in a quoted study in the National Institutes of Health Pub Med website to be effective at increasing free testosterone in the bloodstream in men that had low free testosterone to begin with. No significant increase was noted in men with normal levels of free testosterone. They concluded it might be possible that the effect of zinc supplementation on free testosterone depends on exercise.

Tongkat Ali is a well-known herb from Malaysia that is   15 also known as Malaysian Ginseng. It has been used for centuries as a remedy for male impotence and as a method to increase testosterone and male virility. Studies are mixed on its effectiveness with regard to increasing testosterone.

Raw glandular supplements are reported to increase activity in the specific gland that they correspond to. In other words, testicular glands that are raw and obtained from pigs or cattle are expected to increase the activity of the testes in otherwise healthy human males. This is due to the similarity of the makeup of pigs/cattle and human body systems. There are studies that show the effectiveness of raw glandulars in humans and animals.

Depending on the quality, there may be some hormones in the tissue of the glands which were preserved by the freeze drying process the manufacturers use in producing these glands. This can be helpful to bodybuilders who are looking for raw orchic(testicular) glands to increase their testosterone level. The amount will most likely be a trace and no more, but coupled with the other benefits can be a help.

The supplements listed are to be used as a general guideline and aren't intended to be an exhaustive list of possible testosterone boosters. Science is constantly striving to gain new insight into effective hormone boosters that are both safe and effective at increasing hormone levels in bodybuilders to aid in muscle growth.

There are three forms of strength in a muscle: The raising of weight or eccentric, the holding of a weight motionless or static and the negative or lowering phase. Its important to fully exhaust a muscle in all three strength levels to derive the most benefit. To further clarify, when you are curling a barbell up in the barbell curl you are using the first type; near the top when you are struggling to hold the bar for 10 seconds you are using the second and when you fight the downward descent, you are using the last.

Strength Training Principles

There are some principles which hold true no matter the level of experience of the bodybuilder. They form the basis of effective training programs and must be followed if positive results will be realized.

Specificity

SAID, or specific adaptation to imposed demands means that training should be designed to subject the muscles to exercises done in a manner that leads to the desired results.

For instance, if an advanced bodybuilder wants to build more definition in his physique, in addition to proper diet, will shorten the rest periods between sets of an exercise and use a faster pace in his exercises. If he desires to build more forearm strength, he will use wrist curls and gripping exercises using heavy weights for low reps.

If he desires to build a bigger chest, he will train chest first in all sessions using a moderate rep count, progressive overload, a variation of exercises and intensity techniques and use the proper training frequency.

Progressive Overload

Progressive overload is key to success in weight training and bodybuilding. Without progressive overload there will be little or no gains in mass and strength. Progressive overloading is the act of adding to the weight lifted or increasing the repetitions in an exercise with the same weight.

If you have been using 110 lbs. in the barbell curl for 10 reps, adding 5 lbs to the bar and completing 10 reps or doing 12 reps with 110 lbs is a common way to overload. The aim is to have small increases in weight to avoid the Golgi Tendon limitation as mentioned previously.

Double Progressive Overload

Instead of adding weight to an exercise while using the same rep count, try both increasing the weight and adding additional reps. Since you are increasing the workload on a muscle in two different ways, it is referred to as double progressive overload.

This works well if a light weight is added to the bar or machine. To do this, buy or make micro-loading weight plates, each plate weighing between 5/8-1 ½ lbs. I explain the method to make these in my book, "DR HIT's Ultimate Bodybuilding Guide:Chest."

Individual Specificity

Each bodybuilder has specific needs and goals to help them

develop a better physique. Training programs must be tailored to the individual bodybuilder taking into consideration such factors as experience level, existing strength levels, conditioning, recuperative ability and tolerance to exercise.

Since no one program is optimal for all bodybuilders, beginners must use the knowledge of advanced bodybuilders and books such as the one you're reading to educate themselves or risk years of poor training results.

Variation

If a particular training regimen is used week in and week out for months on end, progress will quickly stagnate and all gains will come to a halt because the body quickly adapts to training demands imposed on it and fights to remain at status quo.

New training routines need to be introduced as well as rep schemes altered and new exercises and techniques used to restart progress. Shocking routines outlined elsewhere in this book are a great way to set the body in motion for new gains.

The Need For High Training Intensity

One of the basic tenets of bodybuilding training is the higher the training intensity is the lower the duration of training must be. As intensity of effort increases a trainee must lower the amount of sets both per muscle group and the overall workout structure. If this isn't done the bodybuilder will overtrain, risk losing muscle, experience a lack of interest in training and will be lethargic during the day.

Just how does one determine the proper intensity level to instigate new muscle growth?

The easy answer to that question is to end a set of an exercise when you hit muscular failure, when no more reps are possible after expending 100% effort. Let's use the overhead barbell press as an example. If we select a weight that allows 10 reps to be completed and no more, the first 5 reps will be pretty easy. The 6th through 8th reps will be moderately hard to complete. The 9th rep will be hard to complete and the 10th will just barely be attainable. As the 11th rep is attempted, the bar will progress up several inches only to begin descent back down to the shoulders. The weight or rep count should be increased slightly at each workout in an attempt to overload the muscle.

Some HIT variables , which are explained in the next section, should be included to take the set past the point of failure to give proper muscle growth stimulus. I really like forced reps, negatives and partials for this purpose.

Many of the variables can be practiced while training alone; some can not. For instance, forced reps typically require a training partner to assist you in completed extra reps at the end of a set but can be done while training alone if one-armed exercises are done with either dumbbells or a cable machine. The same goes for negatives; a training partner is needed if using a barbell, but if a machine, cable or dumbbell is used unilaterally, negatives can be safely done while training alone.

The Danger Of Excessive Training

Most bodybuilders, myself included, absolutely love the feel of training with weights, bands and the like. This can cause one to train with extra sets and exercises. What will eventually happen is the bodybuilder will have lackluster results in the gym, experience the onset of extreme fatigue, and will many times cease training altogether due to frustration.

How do we determine what the ideal set count per body part, total sets per workout, and training frequency is? While there are standard guidelines, the best method to determine this is through trial and error. Each individual is unique in their tolerance to exercise, ability to put forth maximum exertion and recuperate from vigorous exercise.

Of course, another determining factor involved in this is the training protocol used. If a HIT devotee, the overall volume of work will be very low due to the high intensity level. Bodybuilders training using the High Volume protocol will use an amount of training that falls in the range of 8-20 sets for small muscles and 12-25 for larger ones.

Medium volume bodybuilders will use 6-10 sets for small muscles and 10-15 for large muscles.

How often should I train? This is a common question and will be dependent on the natural and built-up recovery ability of the individual bodybuilder. Some trainees have a very 21 high tolerance for training and will rebound very quickly from intense exercise. Others will need a bit longer to be back at 100% while others will need much longer to replenish energy levels and build muscle.

As mentioned previously, it will be necessary to experiment to determine the ideal recovery time for yourself. Pay particular attention to soreness in the muscles,overall energy levels and the level of strength in each workout. If your strength levels haven't either increased or have been reduced, you haven't rested adequately. As a rule of thumb a muscle shouldn't be trained more than once every seven days. If you find yourself in need of additional rest after seven days, try resting for 10 days to see if that is sufficient.

The total days allocated for training shouldn't exceed three times in a given week. With that amount of training you should be at a healthy balance of rest versus work. Remember, training stimulates the muscles to grow but the body actually grows during rest periods. If there isn't adequate rest the body will break down and the muscles won't grow and many times will actually reduce in size.

Limitations To Increased Strength And Muscle Size

There are natural limitations to the level of strength and muscle size that can be achieved with even the best bodybuilding and powerlifting training. These are classified into physiological and psychological. Physiological limitations are the physical attributes of the body that cause restraints on muscle growth and strength.

Poor neuromuscular efficiency severely limits the activation of muscle fibers during an exercise leading to less stimulation of muscle cells and resulting growth. What causes this? Normally the central nervous system sends a signal to the bundles of muscle fibers in the muscle being trained to lift the weight during an exercise. Some people, who are fortunate to have excellent neuromuscular efficiency can lift very heavy weights even though they may have only average muscle mass.

If you've ever attended a powerlifting event, you no doubt witnessed a lifter who looks like he/she didn't even train, lift enormous amounts of weight. This is due to a natural ability to recruit a large amount of muscle fibers to lift very heavy weights.

Practicing the lifts also builds additional neuromuscular efficiency because the body becomes accustomed to executing the lifts. So while there are naturally strong athletes, through practice and training it is possible to improve nerve/muscle efficiency and lift more weight.

Another physical limitation to the lifting of heavy weights are Golgi Tendons. These are nerve sensors which are connected at the point where tendons attach to the muscles. Their job is to determine if the amount of stress to a muscle is too much for the muscle to handle without becoming injured and will send signals to the brain to cease contraction of the muscle to prevent injury.

They do this in conjunction with bands of extrafusal fibers, which are sensors located in the ligaments of joints. These fibers detect the dangerous levels of exertion and send the information to the Golgi Tendons which then forwards this to the brain.

If the amount of stress is too great the sensors' activity increases and the contraction is completely shut down. If you typically bench press 250 pounds for 10 reps but load the bar with 500 pounds, the doubling of weight would cause the Golgi Tendons to send a signal to completely shut down the lift.

To properly increase the load use a weight of 255, just 5 pounds over your normal load and do 10 reps with that. If successful, you will have increased the weight by such a slight amount the Golgi Tendons won't have been stimulated at all. This is an example of the proper method to progressively overload your muscles and continue to make gains.

In the late 1800's, a scientist by the name of Michel Georges discovered a gene he named GDF-8. This gene is responsible for the production of the protein Myostatin, which regulates the amount of muscle mass the body can ultimately develop. In other words, Myostatin determines one's genetic potential for bodybuilding.

There is a Belgian Blue Bull which carries triple the muscle mass that a normal bull does due to almost non-existent amounts of Myostatin. Conversely, bodybuilders that are so-called genetic freaks rippling with almost superhuman muscle mass most likely have the same situation the Belgian Blue Bull does.

While all of this may discourage bodybuilders that have a hard time adding even an ounce of muscle to their frame, there are efforts underway to develop supplements and drugs to inhibit the production of Myostatin in the human body. Novartis Pharmaceuticals has developed a drug, as of the writing of this book, that has been shown to inhibit Myostatin and several supplement companies have done the same.

Muscle size is determined by its length because a muscle is never wider than its length. Take a look at your biceps and note whether there is a large gap where your tendon inserts into your forearm. If there is you don't have great potential for bicep development. If the three heads of your triceps have a large gap between the muscle and elbow, you are limited in muscle size potential.

Muscle density is also a factor. A dense muscle has many more fibers than a less dense one. The denser muscle has many more fibers to recruit to lift weights and grow.

Recovery ability is a definite factor in bodybuilding success. If you are a bodybuilder that requires 10-14 days between workouts for the same muscle you won't have the same training opportunities that one that requires only five days does.

Keep in mind that as you become more advanced you make greater in-roads to your central nervous system, and since your body doesn't become more efficient at removing the   25 waste products that result from intense training, it is very important to give yourself ample time to recover between sessions.

So far we have listed some of the physiological reasons for failure to add new muscle to your physique. Now let me list some of the psychological reasons that could hamper you in your quest for more muscle.

Muscles are capable of delivering incredible power when needed. To demonstrate this, we need to take a look at incidents in which an average built woman lifts a car off her husband who became trapped as a result of being under a car and having the car slip off the jack. How is it possible that she can lift the car off her husband and bodybuilders fail to lift much lighter weights during training?

A typical male's muscles are capable of exerting a force of 140 pounds per square inch and a female 105 pounds per square inch. That equates to a lot of potential power but unfortunately only a small fraction (30%) of that is used during training because our minds are reluctant to allow us to tap into that. We are wired to conserve energy at all costs both physically and mentally.

The reason is all-out bursts of strength like lifting a car off someone completely exhausts our energy reserves, putting us dangerously low in the event another life-threatening situation happens. The key is to constantly challenge ourselves to focus better and push ourselves harder during training to utilize more of our strength reserves.   26

One study showed that 30% more effort was possible when a fight-or-flight stimulus was given four seconds prior to a maximum attempt on a strength measuring device. This is one method to bypass the mental limitations that exist. If you attend a weightlifting or powerlifting meet, you will see many lifters using smelling salts just before a maximum attempt. This clears their head and focuses their concentration on lifting the weight.

Many trainers yell loudly and even slap their lifters in the face to psych them up. This works because it makes the lifter angry and instigates the fight-or-flight response. Short of slapping our training partner, how can we elicit the same positive results?

Some years ago, a doctor by the name of John Zeigler developed a machine called an electronic muscle stimulator, or EMS, that bypasses the existing mental and neuromuscular shortcomings.

It allows an athlete to stimulate almost 100% of the muscle's fibers during a contraction by use of an electric current generated by the machine and delivered via 2-4 pads placed on the skin on either side of the muscle. I have one of these machines and can attest to the effectiveness of its ability to produce a much stronger contraction than I can on my own during training.

The machine isn't practical to use during a workout as it would probably get broken or dropped and the pads would become dislocated. It would be impossible to time the contractions generated by the machine with the contractions from the exercise you would be performing. Therefore, the

EMS is most useful for injury rehab and as a way to add extra stimulation to the muscles after a training session.

Hard bodybuilding training can be intimidating for some and requires focus and strong willpower if you are to be successful. Many new trainees lack the courage or willpower to train with enough intensity to stimulate growth in muscles. Over time, if they are determined enough, experience will enable them to overcome this and succeed. Hang photos of bodybuilders and positive sayings in your home gym, if that's where you train.

If you train in a commercial gym, find training partners or make new friends who are serious with their training to help keep you on the right path and avoid becoming discouraged. Take photos of yourself and keep a dated journal of personal bests in weight used during exercises and statistics of body weight, measurements of muscle size and percentage of body fat and muscle.

Some Training Terms Used In This Manual

To educate yourself on some of the terms used in this manual read the following outline. Many of these may be familiar to you, such as supersets,giant sets and forced reps, because they are used in training routines from bodybuilding magazines.

Forced Reps-These are a great way to propel your sets past the point of momentary muscular failure. Typically bodybuilders end exercise sets when no additional reps are possible. This is called muscular failure, which is great for taxing the muscles sufficiently to stimulate new growth. Due to our body's efficient adaptation abilities, we quickly become accustomed to this level of training and need to change things up by further increasing the intensity of our training.

One of the best ways to do this is to use forced reps. To use this technique it is necessary to train with a partner. I will use the bench press to explain the proper method to use forced reps. Load the bar or machine with a weight that causes failure at 10 reps. As you attempt to complete an eleventh rep and begin to fail, your training partner gives just enough assistance by applying two to three fingers and lifting slightly, allowing you to complete this rep. Continue in this fashion until you have done a total of four additional reps.

Pure Negative Reps-Studies have shown that one of the most effective ways to develop strength and muscle size quickly is to do negative-only reps in your training. There are two distinct portions of a movement, the raising, or positive portion and the lowering, or negative portion. The negative is the strongest zone because the muscle is using the friction of its fibers moving against one another to slow down the lowering of the weight.

I recommend using a weight that is 40% more than is used in a normal set of an exercise. Ideally have a training partner lift the weight and transfer the weight to you at the top of the movement, then lower the weight slowly until you are at 29 the bottom. Repeat.

Negative-Accentuated-These are similar to pure negatives except these can be done without the assistance of a training partner. Lift the weight with both arms, lower it with the left arm first, lift the weight with both arms and lower it using the right arm. It won't be feasible to place the entire weight on one arm or leg but you will be able to transfer most of it. Like the pure negatives, lower the weight slowly to a count of eight.

Negative-Emphasis

This technique has the bodybuilder lifting a weight using a normal cadence but slowing the negative portion down drastically to reap the benefits of the lowering phase. For example, lift the bar during a barbell curl with a two-second count. Instead of lowering the bar using a count of four, lower it using an 8 count. The reduced speed will tax the muscle and cause more micro-damage, leading to a greater rebuild of muscle tissue.

Superslow-In an effort to prevent injuries and increase the intensity of effort during training, Ken Hutchins, an associate of Nautilus inventor Arthur Jones, began using a protocol of 10 seconds lifting and 10 seconds lowering for each rep of an exercise. He found that lowering a weight for 10 seconds allowed a muscle to rest so he revised it to a 4 second negative. Since the ideal time tension for muscle growth is typically 45-60 seconds I recommend doing a total of five reps in each set.

30

Extended Reps-Extended Reps take the concept of

Superslow reps even further. This technique uses one rep to make up the entire set by performing the rep in the following way: Using the chin-up as an example, pull yourself up taking 30 seconds to do so. Pause one second at the top then lower yourself for 30 seconds.

The idea is to use extreme fatigue in the muscle to activate the maximum number of fibers, thereby leading to more gains in muscle and strength. This technique can be used in many exercises to give them a unique action on the muscle. A different method of performing this is to complete the negative zone before the positive one.

Using the chin-up as an example, step up so that you are at the top of the bar and lower yourself down to a count of 30. Pause one second at the bottom before pulling yourself to the top using a count of 30.

Rest-Pause-One of the problems with conventional training is the build-up of lactic acid in the muscle which leads to cessation of a set before the muscles fail on their own. This technique remedies that situation by pausing for ten seconds between reps to allow the blood to flush the lactic acid away before performing the next rep. Because of this, maximum weights can be used for the appropriate time under tension, which is great for building size fast. A typical set performance is as follows:

Machine press-1 x8, max singles with 90-95% of 1rm with 10 second rest periods in-between.

Select a weight on the stack that is near your max single

attempt. Press the machine's arms up to the point prior to lockout, pause one second then return. Rest for 10 seconds then repeat. After the second rep it will be necessary to reduce the weight approximately 10% to facilitate the completion of a third rep. Reduce the weight as needed to complete maximum reps until the desired rep count of 10 is achieved.

Another way to use Rest-Pause is to switch to three rep cycles. Use a weight that maxes you out for three reps. Do three reps, rest for ten seconds then repeat using three rep sequences interspersed with 10 second rests. This allows you to use lighter weights yet gain the benefits associated with elimination of lactic acid build-up.

Static Holds-Using the different techniques outlined here and in my other books allows you to push yourself to and past the limit of muscular failure during your workouts. The goal is to find the best way to maximize the amount of weight used for a given rep goal,striving to constantly increase it and training with the highest level of intensity possible to stimulate new muscle gains. Of utmost importance is safety during this process to allow the bodybuilder to avoid injuries and training downtime.

Static holds are one of the newer HIT variables available and were developed on the premise that since the use of heavy weights assist bodybuilders in increasing intensity of effort, it would be beneficial to maximize the weight with a limited 32 rep scheme.

To do this one loads the bar or weight machine with a weight that is 90-95% of 1RM and lifts the weight into the position where the most muscle fibers are used to hold the weight for 10-20 seconds. Usually this is the point at the top of an exercise just prior to lockout. Or in the case of pull-downs, the point where the bar is at the bottom.

A set consists of a series of holds interspersed with 10 second rest periods. One variation is called "Pyramid Holds." To do this select a weight that is 80% of your 1RM and lift it in position, holding it for 10 seconds. Set the weight down and rest for 10 seconds. Increase the weight by 5% and hold it in position for 10 seconds.

Continue until you have reached your maximum weight. Reduce the weight and hold it for 10 seconds. Continue in this fashion until you have gone down the weight stack. This format eliminates the need to use extremely heavy weights, which can be dangerous and lead to injuries if the hold technique isn't executed properly.

Supersets-These are a mainstay of old-school bodybuilding and have been used by virtually all bodybuilders in their quest for more efficient methods to build muscle. They can be done in a variety of ways but the most common is to group two exercises for the same muscle group and do them one after the other with zero rest in-between. I recommend doing an isolation exercise as your first movement followed by a compound one. What this looks like for chest is: 33

- Pek dek-1x12

- Machine bench presses-1x8

This form of superset training is called pre-exhaust because it isolates the muscle with the first exercise, which primarily trains the target muscle exclusively, then adds a second exercise, which is a compound one, to train the muscle past the point of muscular failure.

Another way to use supersets is to train antagonistic muscles. A great example is an arm routine like the following:

- Concentration curls-1x12

- Triceps press-downs-1x10

- Barbell curls-1x10

- Lying triceps extensions-1x12

The first and third exercises train the biceps muscle while the second and fourth train the triceps. By alternating a biceps exercise with a triceps one, you will get a great pump in each muscle. Studies have shown there is a greater output of strength in each muscle when trained this way. Part of this is due to the amount of blood in the muscle which flushes it with fresh, muscle-building nutrients.

Tri-Sets-These add a third exercise to an existing superset. Like the superset, they are performed by grouping exercises for the working muscle and completing them with no rest in-between. They allow bodybuilders to really blast the muscles and improve aerobic conditioning at the same time.   34 When putting trisets together try and use both isolation and compound exercises in each tri-set so the muscle can be worked by itself and with the assistance of fresh, complimentary muscles.

In the following example the first exercise is an isolation movement while the last two are compound ones.

Here is a sample workout for the back:

- Straight-arm pull-downs-1x12
- Dumbbell rows-1x8
- High rows-1x10

Giant Sets-These are closely related to supersets but instead of using two exercises for each muscle, they group together three or more exercises. These are great for developing a shirt-busting pump as well as hitting the muscle from many different angles. Like supersets, these can be structured by using exercises for one muscle or alternating exercises for opposing muscles.

An example of a giant set for chest is:

- Dumbbell flyes-1x12
- Barbell bench press-1x10
- Machine dips-1x10
- Incline dumbbell bench press-1x10
- Dumbbell decline bench press-1x12

If a bodybuilder desires to train using the opposing muscle group approach the following can be used to train both chest and back:

- Pek dek-1x12

- Nautilus pullovers-1x12

- Barbell bench press-1x10

- Dumbbell rows-1x8

- Decline bench press-1x12

- Barbell deadlifts-1x8

- Bar dips-1x12

- Pull-downs-1x10

I suggest using both methods to add variety to your training. The same holds true as it did in our example above, both the chest and back are stronger when alternated due to the increased pump and greater nervous/muscle stimulation.

You can even group exercises together for the entire body to make up a giant set. This is called circuit training and is very effective at strengthening and conditioning the entire body.

The Workouts

HIT

I will outline effective workouts for each muscle group as well as full body circuit routines to condition and develop the entire body. The exercises are explained thoroughly in other training manuals I've written so won't be elaborated on here. From reading my other books you no doubt realized HIT,   36 or high intensity is my training protocol of choice. This is due to the extensive, and growing research proving its effectiveness at increasing muscle mass and strength in a brief period of time. Brief both in duration of workouts and in the time needed to see results.

This form of training emphasizes brief, intense workouts and focuses on the performance of just enough training volume to elicit maximum muscle growth while avoiding overtraining. Generally one set is done per exercise because logic dictates that if one set of an exercise is done with enough intensity of effort then any additional sets are not only a waste of time but would require pacing yourself to allow completion of the additional sets. This would cause all initial sets to be done with inadequate effort to stimulate new muscle growth.

There are many facets to HIT training and it seems as if new ways to apply this form of training appear everyday. My first book, "DR HIT's Effective High Intensity Variables" is a comprehensive guide to the proper use of many different variables, or training techniques used to increase the intensity of your workouts.

Medium Volume

This type of training is the one most common among non-competitive bodybuilders and is an effective protocol for many trainees. While not as efficient as HIT, it uses moderate intensity and a set count that allows solid training while avoiding overtraining.

Generally referred to as Old School Bodybuilding, it uses 37 routines espoused by many bodybuilders of the 40',50's and 60's. Steroid use was in its infancy among competitive bodybuilders so they had to be conscious of maintaining the proper amount of work for each muscle or risk overtraining.

Set counts for smaller muscle groups falls in the range of 6-10; larger muscles have a range of 8-15. This is excessive from a HIT perspective but allows a low-moderate intensity of effort. While HIT typically uses one working set for each exercise, medium volume exercises are comprised of more than one set.

The bodybuilder paces him/herself to allow the completion of these sets and actively "chases" the pump. This makes the muscle full with blood giving it a feeling of hardness. The size of the muscle increases as a result and research shows this leads to an increase in non-pumped muscle size.

A sample workout for chest is:

- Inclined dumbbell flyes-3x12
- Flat barbell bench press-4x12,10,8,6
- Bar dips-3x10
- Declined dumbbell bench press-3x12,10,8,6

High Volume

This type of training is the one that most professional bodybuilders use. They are able to do this because of their use of steroids and other growth hormones and drugs. These drugs cause a dramatic increase in protein synthesis, which allows a muscle to use a lot more protein than it normally 38 could to build muscle quickly.

Recuperative ability is dramatically increased as well,

allowing the bodybuilder to train longer and more often. If a non-drug user were to train with a pro bodybuilder's regimen, he would quickly overtrain and lose muscle mass. As a result of these conditions, I won't be including high volume routines in this manual.

Types of Training Equipment Used In The Routines

There are many different types of weight training and resistance training equipment available. Not all of them are effective and some are downright dangerous to use. I will be giving you training routines that feature barbells, dumbbells, bands and weight machines. Each of these has specific benefits to their use and some drawbacks. The following information is based on research and personal experience.

Barbells

This is the most popular tool and one that many bodybuilders,weightlifters and powerlifters consider to be the most valuable tool in their training. Simple in concept and design, it is very effective at loading resistance on your muscles, using both isolation and compound exercises. The barbell is great to use for adding muscle bulk with compound exercises, such as the bench press,squat and dead lift. These lifts work large muscle groups, which helps to add muscle to your physique fast, if properly done.

A major drawback with barbell training is the poor mechanical leverage that many of the exercises offer.   39 The best example I can give is the barbell curl. If we take a look at the leverage throughout the exercise it becomes apparent this exercise, while a good muscle builder, has serious flaws in it.

The beginning portion places heavy resistance on the biceps . This increases as the bar moves up until it hits mid-point. Immediately after that the resistance leaves the muscle due to a bad angle and only increases slightly as the bar reaches the top. Unfortunately this allows the biceps to rest while training, which is counter-productive to muscle growth.

All of this being said, we will be using the barbell in our training because of its simplicity and effectiveness for the reasons listed above.

Dumbbells

These are a derivative of barbells and are wonderful free weight tools. They allow a full range of motion on every exercise, and are in reality two separate mini barbells. Maximum weights can be used due to their safety. For example,during the bench press it is common for inexperienced trainees to get "caught" under the bar when failing if not using a spotter. With dumbbells this is impossible; just drop the dumbbells on the floor instead. This is just one example.

If you are training in a public gym there will be a dumbbell rack with a full complement of fixed-weight dumbbells. This is great as it eliminates the necessity of changing the weight during training, which is always a hassle. If you are 40 training in your own home gym and have some money available, I recommend you invest in a sturdy dumbbell rack and a line of fixed dumbbells. A rack is a wonderful space saver and keeps your weights off the floor.

One very effective technique to use dumbbells with is called up-and-down the rack. To do this with standing front lateral raises, grab a pair of dumbbells that are fairly light and do a set of laterals. Set the weights down and grab the next heaviest pair and do a set with those. Continue increasing the weight until you are maxed out. Work your way down the rack in the same way you worked your way up. After this your delts will be burning and pumped to the max. Many exercises are great to use with method.

The only drawback to dumbbells is the same as barbells. Many exercises suffer from poor mechanical leverage, so the resistance fluctuates and allows the muscles to rest at different zones of an exercise.

Bands

These consist of surgical tubes,rubber straps and heavy duty rubber power bands. All three are great training tools and impart slightly different stimulation to the muscles than either free weights or machines. One of the great things about bands is since they are lightweight, they are easy to take with you on vacation so you are able to continue your training program while away.

A great feature is the increase in tension as you extend them which is great for maximum exertion at the point of peak 41 contraction. Unlike free weights there is no issue with bad leverage so they are great to use for virtually any exercise from any angle.

Power bands come in a full range of resistance levels so they are suitable for all but the strongest trainee. They were originally used by powerlifters to add a steadily increasing resistance to the bar as it was being lifted in one of the three power-lifts. This helped them build the explosive power necessary to blast the bar upward during a maximum attempt at a competition meet.

There are many effective ways to train with bands , but I recommend using them in conjunction with other types of equipment. For instance, after training to failure in the machine curl, perform a different form of the curl with a band to build a maximum contraction in the finished position.

An example is as follows:

- Nautilus machine curl-1x12 to failure

- Band concentration curl-1x10 to failure

In this sequence do the first exercise to failure then use a moderate resistance band to complete a set of concentration curls to failure. After ending the set do a series of fast,short, pulsing reps until you are unable to move the band at all. These burn reps are a favorite of mine and are a great way to push your muscles past failure.

Bands can be used to train any muscle group including legs, chest and back. I will explain how to properly complete a new exercise when outlining the workouts.

Weight Machines

Weight machines gained immense popularity when the Nautilus Machines created by Arthur Jones hit the market. Mr. Jones promoted his machines by establishing Nautilus only fitness centers, which focused on his brand of high intensity training. These were comprised of three day per week sessions of full body workouts, where each muscle was trained with two sets -one set of two different exercises to failure. The first exercise was an isolation movement; the second was a compound one. This is a very effective HIT variable called pre-exhaust superset.

To prove his machines were effective at building muscle faster than free weights, Mr. Jones set up the Colorado Experiment in Fort Collins, Colorado, under the supervision of Dr. Elliot Plese in the Colorado State University's Department of Physical Education Laboratory. He trained a 19 year old bodybuilder by the name of Casey Viator who gained a total of 63 pounds of lean muscle mass in less than eight hours of training. The experiment proved how effective both Nautilus machines and High Intensity training was.

After a short time manufacturers by the name of Cybex, Promaxima and others appeared on the scene and the Nautilus Fitness Centers vanished. Arthur Jones sold his Nautilus machines and started a new company with its own line of machines by the name of Med-Ex.   43

These machines, while excellent machines to build muscle, focused on rehabilitation of athletes. The weight stacks were pushed up instead of being pulled up during use, making exercises smoother than other machines.

Pros and Cons of Weight Machines

I like the effect weight machines have on bodybuilding training and have experienced very positive results both in muscle gain and conditioning from them.

There are many different manufacturers of weight machines-some of them produce quality machines and others lack the engineering staff, quality control and market machines that don't effectively train the body. It is extremely important to have a design that uses a proper movement path or you risk injury at worst, and at best, don't receive the proper stimulation of your muscles.

If using a professional gym you should be OK. If you are assembling your own gym at home check online sites such as Craigslist for good used equipment. You'll find good buys and will soon realize heavy duty gym equipment, while very durable,doesn't maintain strong values. Buy a good multipurpose gym to use as your core machine and add pieces to augment it and add variety to your training.

Machines are safe to use as it is impossible to drop weights like it is with free weights. When using the static hold technique, rest-pause and drop sets, machines with selectorized weight stacks allow quick weight change which makes them more effective. Machines are available to train every muscle group using both isolation and compound exercises.

Some bodybuilders, who are die hard free weight advocates, avoid machines with a passion and claim that it is necessary to use only compound free weight exercises to add muscle and strength. While free weights are invaluable tools for adding muscle mass and strength they are only one tool in a bodybuilder's arsenal. As long as the resistance level is high enough to work the muscles hard, machines apply the same stimulation as free weights do.

Because they are engineered with the proper exercise path and offer a cam or other system to alter the resistance placed on the muscle during an exercise, machines are superior for muscle development.

Using the curl as an example, when using a barbell or dumbbell you will hit a sticking point where the leverage causes the bar to stop. Because you are limited to the use of a weight that allows you to move the bar past this point you are not able to add weight until you have gotten strong enough to power past this sticking point.

With a properly cammed weight machine you will be able to complete the exercise because the cam alters the resistance throughout the movement to follow the biceps strength curve. To see this clearly look at an older Nautilus machine's cam and you will notice that it is an odd shape and the thickness varies throughout. The thinner the cam the easier it is to lift the weight. Conversely the thicker the cam is the harder it 45 is to lift the weight.

As for cons of weight machines, the only one I can think of is since they isolate muscles they sometimes limit the body's functional movement. This questionable negative feature can be easily overcome by training with compound exercises which involve a large amount of muscle groups.

Weight Machines' Ability to Allow Use of a Varied Amount of Training Techniques

Since machines allow precise control of exercise movement, they are ideally suited to use with such training techniques as forced reps,negative reps,super-slow reps and the like. If we compare the use of machines with free weights during negative reps it is easy to see how much safer machines are.

Using the flat bench press as an example, during a free weight bench press the bar would be raised mostly with the training partners' effort. The weight would be transferred to the bodybuilder who then lowers the bar slowly, usually to a count of eight. This is repeated until the bodybuilder is unable to control the downward movement of the bar.

If this was duplicated on a machine the weight would again be lifted by the training partners who would transfer the weight to the bodybuilder. As the bodybuilder continues with the set and becomes increasingly fatigued, the weight descends more quickly. The worst that could happen is the weights could come crashing down on the stack. There is no way the machine's arms could pin the bodybuilder unlike free weights.

Machines are also wonderful to use for forced reps because of the ease in applying a small amount of pressure to the movement arm to allow rep completion. The motion tends to be smoother lending itself to better control of the exercise.

Nautilus used to produce machines called Omni machines. The Biceps and Triceps machines allow you to use your legs to push down on a footplate to bring the machine arms to the top of the exercise. This allows you to train with pure negatives without a training partner. Unfortunately Nautilus no longer manufactures these.

Smith machines are basically a combination of free weights and machines. Most Smith machines are comprised of a barbell attached to a vertical sliding tube that moves along a tight track. There is a very good safety feature that applies a brake if the bar is dropped to immediately stop the bar's movement, preventing injury to the lifter. Hooks are attached to the bar allowing placement of the bar anywhere on the exercise's path.

These machines are often criticized for the strict exercise path they use which can influence the form of lifts like deadlifts, squats, presses and bench presses. Nevertheless, these machines are very safe and are very useful training tools.

Intensity of Effort Needed To Stimulate New Muscle Growth

One of the most confusing principles in bodybuilding is the intensity of effort needed to instigate new muscle growth, 47 or hypertrophy.

Many bodybuilders complete their training sets one to two

reps before hitting muscular failure. They are interested in generating a strong muscle pump which is effective at stimulating muscle growth due to the infusion of nutrients and hydraulic pressure in the muscle. Studies have shown this to stimulate the increase of both Sarcoplasmic fluid and enlargement of muscle cells. There is a possibility of an increase in the number of muscle cells called Hyperplasia. I say possibility as there isn't any definitive proof of this.

To stimulate new muscle growth it is necessary to inflict minor damage to the muscle fibers. Hard training causes micro-tears in the muscle fibers which causes inflammation of the muscle. The body overcompensates if the damage is adequate and not only repairs the damage to the muscle but adds additional growth. The question then is "What level of intensity is needed to inflict enough damage for muscle growth?"

Studies have shown that while moderate intensity stimulates growth, maximum growth occurs when intensity is at or near 100%. To make sure you are at this level finish all or most of your sets when you are unable to complete any additional reps. This is referred to as muscular failure.

The rule of thumb to follow is: the higher the intensity of effort the lower the training volume must be to prevent overtraining. This is very important to keep focused on because of the temptation to add sets. Many bodybuilders 48 feel that if "x" amount of sets are good, then more sets would be better. This almost always leads to the opposite of what is desired: low energy and muscle loss due to overtraining.

As stated previously, I am an advocate of High Intensity Training but do respect others that desire to train with decreased intensity and a slightly higher set count and will be offering training routines for this form of training as well.

The Training Routines

Medium Volume-Moderate Intensity

Important Notes

- **Use good form in all exercises to prevent injury and to yield better results**
- **Warm up completely by using light weights on the compound exercise for the muscle group being trained**
- **Rest 2-3 minutes between exercises/sets unless indicated otherwise**

Legs

Squats in Smith Machine-5x15,12,10,8,6

Load the bar with a moderately heavy weight. Use a foam pad on the bar if desired for extra comfort. Do 15 reps for the first set stopping 2-3 reps before failure. Rest for two minutes before increasing the weight and doing 12 reps for the second set. Finish by doing the remaining sets, using two minute rest periods between sets. The last set should have a weight   49 sufficient to cause you to end the set at failure.

Leg lunges-3x15,12,10

Use a pair of moderately weighted dumbbells. Being careful

to maintain balance, take a deep step forward with your left leg. Bend down into a deep stance, pause for a second then return. Repeat with the right leg. End the set at 15 reps which should be 2-3 reps prior to failure. Rest 1.5-2 minutes before reducing the dumbbell weight and do a second set. Continue until you have completed a third set of 10 reps to failure.

Leg extensions-3x15,12,10

Use a moderate weight for the first set, ending it 2-3 reps before failure. Increase the weight slightly and complete the second set. End the last set at failure.

Chest

Inclined dumbbell flyes-3x12

Using an inclined bench and a pair of moderately weighted dumbbells, complete three sets of dumbbell flyes. The final set should end at failure.

Flat bench presses-4x12,10,8,6

Beginning with a set of 12 reps using a moderate weight, do a total of four sets. After each set increase the weight slightly. The final set of 6 reps should end at failure.

Bar dips-2x8-10

Add weight via a dip belt if needed and do two sets of 8-10 reps. The last set should end at failure.

Decline bench flyes-2x12

Use a bench with a deep decline. Using moderately weighted 'bells do a total of two sets,the last one ending at failure.

Back

Nautilus or other machine pullovers-3x15,12,10

After every set increase the weight slightly until hitting failure on the final set. Make sure to grip the pullover bar of the machine only slightly as all of the effort should pass through your elbows onto the pads of the machine. Get a full stretch at the beginning while inhaling deeply and exhale as you bring the machine's arms down in front of you, ending at your lower abdomen.

Dumbbell rows-4x12,10,8,6

I prefer to use dumbbells for these because you get a nice stretch at the beginning of the movement. The stretch helps to activate more muscle fibers, increasing your strength throughout the exercise. With each set increase the weight slightly until you end the final set at failure.

Seated cable pull-downs-3x12,10,8

Use a bar attachment where your hands are spaced about 18 inches apart with your hands facing each other. This is the natural position for your lats to work most efficiently. Most bodybuilders use a wide spacing on a lat bar with the palms facing forward with the false belief that this stretches the lats more than a close grip. The idea is that since a wide grip is being used the lats are stretched more. The lats are best 51 stretched with a narrow grip because the range of motion is increased.

Standing cable high rows-3x10

Stand in front of a cable machine with a two-handed strap attached. Get a full stretch at the beginning and pull the handles up high and straight in toward your throat. Pause one second then return the handles to the start position. This exercise works the rhomboid muscles in your upper back and is a great way to thicken them. Do a total of three sets of 10 reps ending the final set near failure.

Machine back extensions-2x15

Select a moderate weight after adjusting the machine for size and extend your upper torso back with a steady motion until parallel with the floor. Repeat. End the final set at failure.

Shoulders

Seated side dumbbell raises-2x12

Do these seated to reduce the chance of momentum. Begin with the dumbbells at your sides and raise them using a smooth motion until they are shoulder height. Pause for one second before lowering. The second set should end one rep before failure.

Seated front raises-2x12

Do these seated for the same reason. Begin with the dumbbells in front of you at leg level. Raise them until they are in front of you at shoulder height. Pause one second before lowering them. Repeat.

Standing barbell presses-4x12,10,8,6

Load the bar with a moderate weight and complete the first set of 12 reps. Make sure to use good form with no hitch or momentum to prevent injury and keep all of the tension on the delts. For the second set reduce the weight on the bar and complete 10 reps. Complete the last two sets the same way, finishing the last set at failure.

Traps

Shoulder shrugs-3x10,8,6

Use a pair of dumbbells or a barbell for this exercise. A machine with a bar handle may also be used. Using a normal two-handed grip and locked arms, shrug your shoulders up to your ears squeezing hard at the top. Pause one second then return. Rest 2 minutes between sets and take all sets to one rep before failure.

Upright rows-3x12

Use a pair of dumbbells for this exercise. Using smooth form bring the weights straight up to shoulder height. Squeeze your traps hard at the top, pause for one second then return to the start position. Take all sets near failure, resting two minutes between sets.

Biceps

Barbell curls

4x12,10,8,6

Load the bar with a moderate weight and complete the first set. Continue with the second set after resting for two minutes. The final set should be to failure.

Preacher curls-3x10

Use a weight that takes you near failure on all sets. This is accomplished by reducing the weight about 10% after each set. Rest two minutes between sets and get a good stretch at the beginning of the exercise to increase your strength.

Lying incline bench curls-3x10

These are great because they force you to use good form throughout. Use a bench set at a steep incline. Grab a pair of dumbbells, lie face down and using good form, curl them up to face level. Pause one second before returning the weight to the bottom. The last set should end one rep before failure.

Palms-facing cable pull-downs-3x10

Select a moderate weight on the stack,use a palms-facing grip and pull the handle down to your upper abdomen. Attempt to focus the effort on your biceps and off your back as much as you can to make this more effective. End the last set close to failure.

Triceps

Standing triceps push-downs-3x10

Select a moderate weight and attach a two-hand rope or double handled triceps bar to the cable. Stand or sit in front of the machine with your elbows locked at your side and your hands against your chest. Push the handle straight down until the handles are at thigh level. You should not lock 54 out on this movement to keep the pressure on your triceps. Reduce the weight 10% for each consecutive set, resting 1.5 minutes between sets.

Lying triceps extensions(scullcrushers)-3x10

Use a pair of moderately heavy dumbbells and a flat bench. While lying face up on the bench, lower the weights to the bench just above your head. Pause one second before extending them overhead, ending just before lockout. Repeat for a total of three sets of 10 reps. All three sets should end 1-3 reps prior to failure.

Close-grip bench presses-4x12,10,8,6

Use a barbell and a flat bench for this exercise. Space your hands 18" apart, bring the weight down to mid-chest and pause one second before pressing it to the point just prior to lockout. Take each set 1-2 reps before failure,reducing the weight 10% and resting two minutes between sets.

Forearms

Wrist roll-ups-1x5 roll-ups

Use a hand held wrist roller or one mounted on the gym wall. Clip a moderate weight onto the end of the cord and unwind it. Hold the roller at shoulder height and use both hands to roll the cord up until the weight is touching the roller. Carefully release the weight to allow the cord to completely unwind. Repeat until you have completed a total of 5 roll-ups.

Abs and Obliques

Stomach crunches on machine-3x20

Use a moderate weight and complete three sets using a smooth movement. Its important to use enough weight to strengthen the ab muscles while avoiding thickening the waist.

Leg raises-3x20

Lie on a flat bench and raise your legs from a flat position until they are 3 feet above the bench. In the beginning use bent knees and progress to straight legs as your abs become stronger. Don't use weight on these to limit growth of the ab muscles. The idea is to tone, strengthen and increase muscle but limit growth to avoid thickening the waist.

If desired you may add a couple of sets to your workout by doing a couple of extra sets of the exercises or add an additional exercise of two sets. Be very careful not to go overboard or you risk overtraining. Train each muscle one to two times per week.

After a couple of months substitute other exercises from the list at the end of this book. This keeps your training fresh and keeps your body "guessing" as to what training you are going to subject it to. The body is very good at adapting to workloads so it is necessary to change your workout program often if you want to continue improving.

Expanded Training Routines-MVT (Medium Volume Training)

I gave examples of workouts at the discussion of each different technique but I am now going to list a series of training routines for each of the major bodybuilding protocols beginning with Medium Volume, or MVT.

Chest

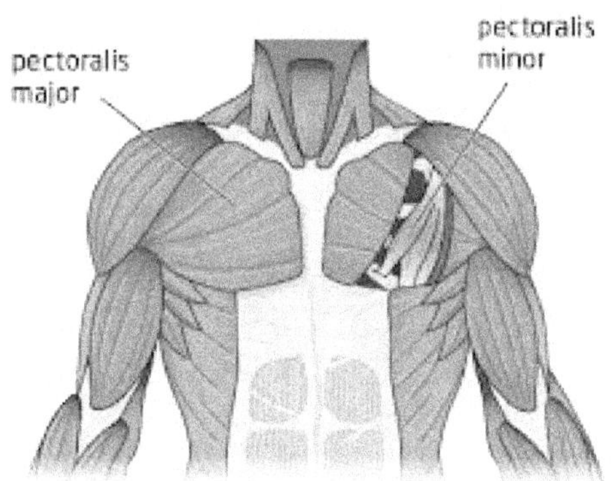

The chest anatomy includes the pectoralis major, pectoralis minor and the serratus anterior. Learn about each of these muscles, their locations, functional anatomy and exercises for them.

Function of the Chest Muscles

The chest is part of a larger group of "pushing muscles" found in the upper body. The chest, as part of this group, enables you to perform pushing actions such as the barbell bench press.

The pectoralis major is a large, fan-shaped muscle and makes up the majority of the chest's muscle mass. It originates at your clavicle, ribs, and sternum, and inserts into the upper portion of your humerus (upper arm bone from elbow to shoulder.)

58

The pectoralis major helps flex the shoulder joint and moves your arm toward and across your chest. When training your pecs you'll likely notice that your shoulders and triceps also benefit.

The pectoralis minor is a thin, triangular muscle that is found underneath the pectoralis major. It attaches at the 3rd, 4th and 5th rib, and reaches to the scapula (shoulder blade.) Its job is to help pull the shoulder forward and down.

The serratus anterior, although not truly part of the chest anatomy, is commonly grouped as part of the chest muscle group because it attaches near the pectorals on the ribs. It's functions are moving the scapula forward and upward.

The Workouts

#1-Standard set

- Flat bench press-6x12,10,8,6,6,4
- Incline bench press-4x12,10,8,5
- Decline dumbbell flyes-4x10
- Low cable crossovers-3x10

Use a barbell or a set of dumbbells for the bench presses (incline and flat). Use a decline bench and a pair of dumbbells for the decline bench presses. The cable crossovers may be done unilaterally or with two pulleys at the same time.

Set the handles at a low position and bring the handles up at an angle. Do the exercises using consecutive sets with   59 1.5 minutes rest between. In other words, do all six sets of flat   bench presses before progressing to the incline bench presses. End all sets one rep before failure.

#2-Standard set

- Pek dek-4x10

- Seated machine dips-5x15,12,10,8,6

- Incline machine bench presses-3x12,10,8

- Dumbbell bench pullovers-3x12

Use a standard pek dek machine for the first exercise. Use a smooth motion throughout, pause for one second at the top and squeeze your pecs hard. Use a seated dip machine for the second making sure to lean forward to accent the chest and take most of the load off your triceps.

For the last exercise, sit in front of a flat bench on the side. As you inhale deeply, lift a moderately heavy dumbbell overhead with arms slightly bent and lower it down over the bench behind you. Exhale as you return the dumbbell overhead. Repeat. Rest 1.5 minutes between sets and end them one rep before failure.

#3-Standard set

- Decline dumbbell bench press -5x12,10,8,6,12

- Flat dumbbell flyes-3x12

- Incline cable flyes-3x10

- Standing bar dips-4x15,12,10,8

Rest 1.5 minutes between sets. Use solid standing dip bars, leaning forward to accent the chest instead of triceps and use a dip belt to add weight if necessary. End all sets one rep before failure.

#4-Standard set

- Alternating cable crossovers(high)-4x15

- Standing bar dips-3x12

- Push-ups with handles-3x12

- Flat bench cable flyes-3x10

- Decline dumbbell bench press-4x12,10,8,6

All sets should end one rep before failure. Rest 1 minute between sets to build up the pump in your chest muscles.

#5 Standard Set

- Band crossovers-one-handed high-3x12

- Decline bench dumbbell flyes-3x10

- Flat barbell bench press-5x12,10,8,8,6

- Standing bar dips-4x12,10,8,8

- Nautilus pullover-3x15

This routine adds bands, a very valuable tool to use in your training. A great feature of bands are the negative resistance they provide and the gradual increase in resistance during the positive portion of an exercise.

This causes the heaviest resistance at the point of maximum contraction, which is a perfect way to activate the majority of fibers in a muscle. All sets of each exercise should be completed before moving on to the next one. Rest 1-2 minutes between exercises.

#6 Standard Set

- Incline barbell bench press-7x15,12,10,8,8,12,15
- Machine dips-4x12,10,8,6
- Flat dumbbell bench press-6x12,10,8,8,6,12
- Pek dek-3x15

All sets should end 1-2 reps before failure. We begin with a light weight on the incline press, work our way up in weight then down again, increasing the reps. This works the exercise using various rep ranges which is good for training the muscle for both strength and size.

The dips begin with a fairly light weight; as the weight is increased the reps decrease accordingly. The first set of the dumbbell bench press begins with light weight, weight is increased then decreased to alter the rep range. I like using varying rep ranges to stimulate muscle growth. The high reps in the pek dek are used to flush nutrient-rich blood into the chest to give it raw materials to grow and increase the Sarcoplasmic fluid in the muscle. Lower reps are used to build power and size by thickening the pectoral's muscle fibers.

#1-Superset

- Dumbbell incline flyes-3x12
- supersetted with
- Machine incline bench press-3x8
- Low pulley cable crossovers-3x15
- supersetted with

- Dumbbell decline bench press-3x8

- Dumbbell pullovers-3x15

- supersetted with

- Standing bar dips-3x8

This superset program for chest totals out at 18 sets. There should be no rest between exercises in the superset and 2 minutes between each superset. In other words, do one cycle of incline flyes followed by one set of machine incline press, rest two minutes then repeat until a total of three cycles have been completed.

Do the second superset in the same fashion after a one minute rest. The final superset consists of dumbbell pullovers and bar dips. All sets should end one to two reps before failure.

#2-Superset

- Flat bench dumbbell flyes-3x12

- supersetted with

- Weighted push-ups with handles-3x12

- Decline flyes-3x12

- supersetted with

- Machine decline bench press-3x10

- Mid-pulley cable crossovers alternating-3x12

- supersetted with

- Incline dumbbell bench press-3x12,10,8

Do this superset like the first, ie., no rest between exercises, 2 minutes rest between supersets and end all sets 1-2 reps shy of failure.

#3-Superset

- Decline dumbbell bench press-3x12,10,8
- supersetted with
- Flat dumbbell bench press-3x12,10,8
- Incline dumbbell bench press-3x12,10,8
- supersetted with
- machine dips-3x12,10,8

This superset concentrates all efforts on the entire chest structure beginning with decline work, which trains the entire chest but focuses on the lower pectorals. The flat bench concentrates on the mid area and the inclines apply extra stimulation to the upper pecs.

#1-Giant Set

- Push-ups on handles-1x15
- Flat bench barbell bench press-1x8
- Incline dumbbell flyes-1x12
- Incline dumbbell bench press-1x10
- Decline dumbbell bench press-1x8
- Decline dumbbell flyes-1x12
- Low pulley cable crossovers-1x25

This giant set covers all bases, flat,incline and decline work and finishes with a good isolation exercise, low pulley cable crossovers. The high reps used are meant to build an incredible pump in the pecs, which flushes them with blood and nutrients.

Not only does the body use these raw materials to build new muscle but the hydraulic pressure which results from the extra blood in the muscle causes trauma to the muscle fibers stimulating them to grow. Each exercise has one set and all exercises should be done one right after another with no rest in-between. After resting for 2-3 minutes a second giant set can be done. If desired a third can be done after an additional 2 minute rest.

#2-Giant Set

- Pek dek-1x15

- Cable crossovers high pulley-1x12

- Incline dumbbell flyes-1x10

- Decline dumbbell flyes

- Nautilus pullovers-1x15

- Machine dips-1x8

- Flat machine bench press-1x6

- Decline dumbbell bench press-1x8

This giant set is designed around the performance of isolation exercises during the first five exercises and compound ones for the last three. All three sectors of chest training are covered: flat,incline and decline.

Different rep ranges are used to stimulate the muscle's various fiber types-fast twitch,slow twitch and hybrids of the two. The low rep sets build strength by working the myofibrillars (muscle fibers) and the higher ranges build a nice pump to get a lot of blood into the muscle, which flushes it with muscle-building nutrients to help it grow.

Chest Routines of Professional Bodybuilders

Lee Haney-Multiple Winner Mr. Olympia

- Bench presses-5x8
- Incline Barbell Bench Press-4x8
- Flat bench flyes-4x10
- cable crossovers-3x10

Rich Gaspari-Mr. Olympia Top Competitor

- Incline dumbbell bench press-7x8-10
- Dumbbell bench press-4x8-10
- Incline dumbbell flyes-4x8-10

Robby Robinson-Mr. Universe Winner

- Incline dumbbell bench press-5x8-10
- Barbell bench press to neck-4x8-10
- Bar dips-4x10-15
- Flat bench flyes-4x8-10

Danny Padilla-Mr. Universe Winner

- Barbell flat bench press-5x12
- Flat bench flyes-5x12
- Incline barbell bench press-5x12
- decline barbell bench press-5x12
- Dumbbell pullovers-5x12
- supersetted with
- Cable crossovers-5x12

Frank Zane-Mr. Olympia Multiple Winner

- Flat bench press-5x6-15
- Incline dumbbell bench press-3x6-20
- Decline dumbbell flyes-3x8-10
- Dumbbell pullovers-3x10

Lou Ferrigno-Mr. Universe/Incredible Hulk

- Flat bench press-7x6-15
- Barbell incline bench press-5x6-10
- Barbell decline bench press-5x6-10
- Flat dumbbell flyes-5x10-12
- Dumbbell pullovers-3x15
- supersetted with
- Cable crossovers-3x10-15

Arnold Schwarzenegger-Mr. Olympia Multiple Winner

- Bench press-5x6-10

- Machine incline bench press-5x6-10
- Bar dips-5x10-15
- Flat dumbbell flyes-5x8-12
- Dumbbell pullovers-5x10-15
- Cable crossovers-5x8-12

Ron Teufel-Mr. USA

- Bench press-7x6-12
- supersetted with
- Dumbbell pullovers-7x10-12
- Machine incline bench press-5x8
- supersetted with
- Decline dumbbell bench press-5x8
- Barbell incline bench press-5x8
- supersetted with
- Cable crossovers-5x10

Boyer Coe-Mr. Universe

- Machine incline bench press-4x8
- Pek dek-4x8
- Vertical machine bench press-4x8
- Incline machine flyes-4x8

Franco Columbu-Mr. Olympia Winner

- Bench press-7x6-8

- Incline barbell bench press-4x6-10

- Flat bench dumbbell flyes-3x8-12

- supersetted with

- Bar dips-3x10-15

Back

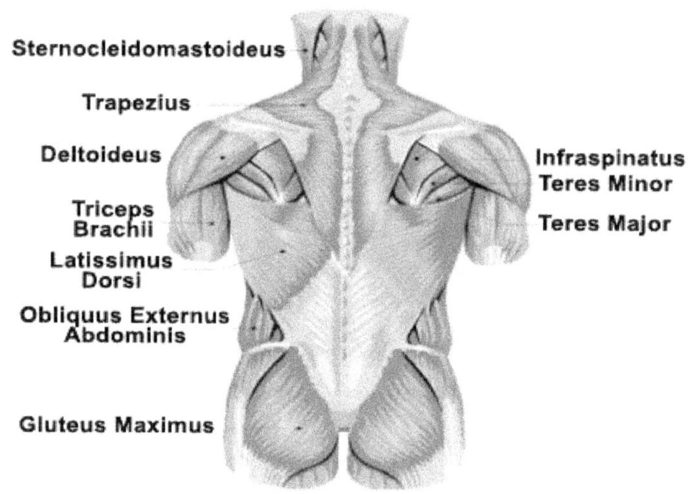

The back is made up of three sections, resembling triangular segments of a pie.

The upper back is made up of large triangular-shaped muscle called the trapezius, which originates along the upper spine from the skull down to the last rib. The upper fibers of the trapezius (in the neck) attach to the outer tip of the shoulder on the clavicle, acromion, and scapula.

The middle and lower fibers of the trapezius (in the upper back) attach to the scapula (shoulder blade). The upper traps elevate the scapula to shrug the shoulder abduction. The middle traps retract the scapula, pulling the shoulders backward; the lower traps depress the scapula downward.

Beneath the trapezius are three muscles that anchor the scapula to the spine: the levator scapulae, rhomboid major, and rhomboid minor. The levator scapulae muscles assist the upper traps to elevate the scapula. The rhomboid muscles work with the middle traps to retract the scapula. These scapular retractor muscles lie under the trapezius and add muscular thickness to the upper back.

The middle back consists of the latissimus dorsi, a large fan-shaped muscle that arises from the lower half of the spinal column and the rear ridge of the pelvic bone (posterior iliac crest). From its large origin, the latissimus converges into a bandlike tendon that attaches to the upper humerus (next to the tendon of the pectoralis major). When the latissimus dorsi contracts, movement takes place at the shoulder joint.

The latissimus dorsi pulls the upper arm downward and backward. The latissimus also pulls the arm in against the side of the body (adduction). The lower back is made up of the erector spinae (or sacrospinalis) muscles that run alongside the entire length of the spinal column.

In the lumbar region, the erector spinae split into three columns: the iliocottalis, longissimus, and spinalis. These muscles are the base of strength in the lower back that stabilize the spine and extend the torso, arching the spine backward.

The trapezius and latissimus dorsi are concerned primarily with movements of the shoulder and arm. It is the sacrospinalis muscles that cause movements of the spine and torso.

Back Routines
#1-Standard Sets

- Dumbbell pullover-3x15
- Barbell Rows-4x12,10,8,6
- High pulley rows-3x10
- Dumbbell shoulder shrugs-3x12,10,8
- End barbell rows-4x10

This routine begins with an exercise that I use in both chest and back routines because it ties in the two areas due to the work it effects on the rib cage for chest and lats for back. The barbell rows are a power builder, able to pack mass on the back quickly. The high pulley rows are great for massing up the rhomboids of the upper back. Dumbbell shoulder shrugs work the traps, which I consider to be a "tie-in" muscle for the shoulders and back.

End barbell rows are a variation of barbell rows but since you are rowing the weight on the end of a barbell instead of either end, they allow the use of heavier weights. End all sets one rep before failure.

#2-Standard Sets

- Seated machine rows-3x10,8,6
- Seated pull-downs-4x12
- Seated reverse pek dek (reverse flye)-3x10
- End barbell rows-4x10,8,8,6
- High pulley rows-3x10

Use a seated row machine for the first exercise. Each brand of machine has their own handle configurations so use one with a comfortable grip. Use a moderate weight for the first set and increase the weight slightly as you go down on reps. Seated pull-downs should be done with a bar that's 24" long with handles that have a palms-facing grip as they give the best grip for training the lats.

Many bodybuilders use a wide grip for pull-downs with a mistaken conclusion that to develop wide lats you need to use a wide grip. The truth is the lats have a greater range of motion when using a medium grip.

There are machines designed for the reverse flye but a pek dek can be used. Sit facing the opposite way you would for a pek dek flye. With slightly bent arms, bring the machine arms back in an arc until they are parallel. The other exercise shave already been described. End all sets one rep before failure.

#1 Superset 73
- Reverse machine fly-3x10
- supersetted with
- dumbbell rows-3x10,8,6
- Stiff-arm pull-downs-3x12
- supersetted with
- Medium-grip pull-downs-3x8
- Nautilus pullovers-3x12
- supersetted with
- High pulley rows-3x10

This superset routine groups isolation exercises with compound ones. The first exercise, an isolation one, "wears down" the back muscles, while the second one, a compound exercise, finishes the muscles off by adding assistive muscles, which are fresh, to exhaust the back beyond what would normally be possible with a typical bodybuilding routine.

Stiff arm pull-downs are done as follows: Lock your arms on a straight bar which is attached to a cable at waist height and pull the bar down until it is against the thighs. Squeeze the lats hard at the bottom for one second then return to the top. Repeat.

#2 Superset
- Barbell row-5x12,10,8,6,6
- supersetted with
- Seated medium -grip pull-downs-5x12,10,8,8,6
- End barbell row-5x10,8,8,8,6
- supersetted with
- Barbell deadlifts-5x10,8,8,6,4

This superset program is designed to quickly build mass and power into your back muscles. All sets should use a weight as heavy as possible and end one rep before failure.

#1 Giant Set
- End barbell row-1x8
- Dumbbell rows-1x10
- Nautilus pullover-1x12
- Reverse flyes-1x10
- Stiff-arm pull-downs-1x12
- Seated medium-grip pull-downs-1x8

- Dumbbell shoulder shrugs-1x6
- High rows-1x10

This giant set begins with two compound exercises, adds three isolation exercises and finishes with three compound ones. This is a good blend of exercises to use for back training because it uses exercises that work all areas of the back except the lower back. For that we'll do the following:

- Back machine extensions -1x12
- Roman chair hyper-extensions-1x15

If you are advanced do a second giant set after resting for 2-3 minutes.

#2 Giant Set
- Deadlifts-1x8
- Seated cable rows-1x10
- Seated cable pull-downs-1x10
- Nautilus pullovers-1x12
- Reverse flyes-1x12
- High rows-1x8
- Upright rows-1x8
- One-arm low cable rows-1x8
- Roman chair hyper-extensions-1x12
- Stiff-legged deadlifts-1x8

This giant set uses three compound exercises in the beginning and adds four isolation exercises before finishing with a set of one-arm cable rows. If advanced, feel free to do a second giant set once you have rested 2-3 minutes.

Back Routines of Top Bodybuilders

Lee Haney-Mr. Olympia Multiple Winner

- Barbell bent rows-5x6-12
- Front lat pull-4x8-10
- Seated pulley rows-4x8-10
- Dumbbell shrugs-4x10-15

Arnold Schwarzenegger-Mr. Olympia Multiple Winner

- Wide-grip front chins5x8-10
- Pull-downs behind neck-5x8-10
- Barbell bent-over rows-5x8-10
- T-bar rows-5x8-10
- Seated cable rows-5x8-10

Samir Bannout-Mr. Olympia Winner

- Pull-downs-3x15-20
- Seated cable rows-4x8-15
- Barbell rows-4x8-15
- Front chins-4x8-12

Sergio Olivia-Mr Olympia Winner

- Wide-grip chins-6x10
- Close-grip chins-5x10
- Wide grip pull-downs-4x6-8
- supersetted with
- Close-grip pull-downs-4x6-8
- Wide-grip cable rows-4x6-8
- supersetted with
- Close-grip cable rows-4x6-8
- Wide-grip pull-downs-4x6-8
- supersetted with

- Narrow-grip pull-downs-4x6-8
- Deadlifts-4x6-8
- supersetted with
- Good mornings-4x6-8

Frank Zane-Mr. Olympia Winner
- Top deadlifts-5x8-10
- Behind neck pull-downs-4x10-12
- Lat pull-downs-4x10-12
- Seated cable rows-4x10-12
- One-arm dumbbell rows-4x10-12

Tim Belknap-Mr. America
- Wide-grip chins-2x10
- Wide-grip pull-downs-3x12-15
- Seated Wide-grip cable rows-3x12-15
- Narrow-grip seated cable rows-3x12-15
- Nautilus pullovers-3x10-12
- Stiff-legged deadlifts-3x10-12
- Hyper-extensions-3x15-25

Lou Ferrigno-Mr. Universe
- Behind-neck chins-5x10-15
- Close-grip barbell rows-5x8-10
- Front chin-ups-5x8-10
- Seated cable rows-5x8-10
- Close-grip pull-downs-5x8-10
- Barbell shrugs-5x10-15

Chris Dickerson-Mr. Olympia
- Front chins-5x10-15
- One-arm dumbbell row-6x8-10
- Behind-neck pull-downs-4x8-10

- One-arm cable rows-4x8-10
- Seated cable rows-4x8-10

Legs
Anatomy

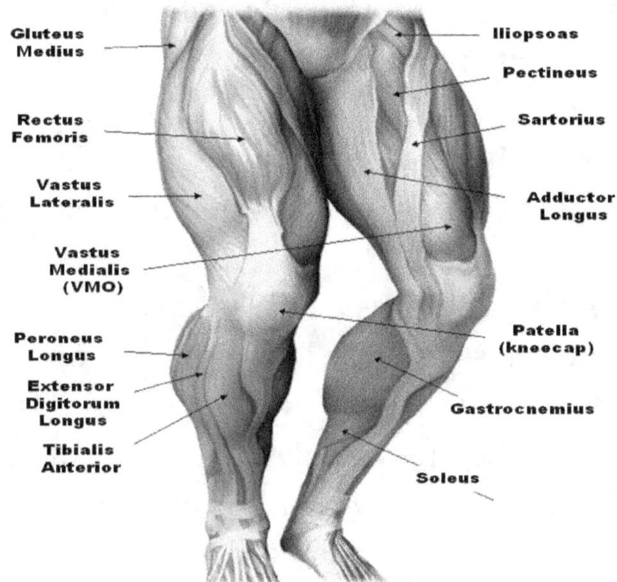

Most of the muscles in the leg are long muscles, giving 79 them the capacity to stretch large distances. As the muscles contract and relax they move skeletal bones, creating movement of the body. Smaller muscles help the larger muscles, stabilize joints, rotate joints, and assist with other fine-tuned movements.

The largest muscle masses in the leg are present in the thigh and the calf.

The **quadriceps** are the strongest and leanest muscles in the body. These four muscles at the front of the thigh are the major extensors of the knee. They are:

•**Vastus lateralis**: On the outside of the thigh, this is the largest of the quadriceps. It extends from the top of the femur to the kneecap.

•**Vastus medialis**: This teardrop-shaped muscle of the inner thigh attaches along the femur and down to the inner border of the kneecap.

•**Vastus intermedius**: Between the vastus medialis and the vastus lateralis at the front of the femur, it is the deepest of the quadriceps.

•**Rectus femoris**: This muscle attaches to the kneecap. Of the four quadriceps muscles it has the least affect on flexing the knee.

The **hamstrings** are three muscles at the back of the thigh that affect hip and knee movement. They begin under the gluteus maximus behind the hipbone and attach to the tibia at the knee. They are:

•**Biceps femoris**: This long muscle flexes the knee. It begins in the thigh area and extends to the head of the fibula near the knee.

•**Semimembranosus**: This long muscle extends from the pelvis to the tibia. It extends the thigh, flexes the knee, and helps rotate the tibia.

•**Semitendinosus**: This muscle also extends the thigh and flexes the knee.

The calf muscles are pivotal to movement of the ankle, foot, and toes. Some of the major muscles of the calf include:

•**Gastrocnemius (calf muscle)**: One of the large muscles of the leg, it connects to the heel. It flexes and extends the foot, ankle, and knee.

•**Soleus**: This muscle extends from the back of the knee to the heel. It is important in walking and standing.

•**Plantaris**: This small, thin muscle is absent in about 10 percent of people. The gastrocnemius muscle supersedes its function.

Leg Routines

#1 Standard Sets

- Leg extensions-4x15
- Leg press-6x10-15
- Sissy squats-3x15
- Lying leg curls-3x15
- Stiff-legged deadlifts-3x12
- Standing calf raises-4x12-15
- Seated calf raises-3x12-20

During leg extensions flex the muscles hard at the point of full extension for one second before returning to start the next rep. While doing the leg press avoid locking out the legs on most reps to keep the tension on the muscles. Sissy squats are done by holding on to a vertical bar and lowering yourself down while leaning back. Your heels will come off the floor if you are going low enough and leaning back properly. Using pure leg power, push yourself back up until upright.

During lying leg curls pull the machine arm up at the top and squeeze your hamstrings hard for one second before lowering the weight back down. Stiff-legged deadlifts are done like standard deadlifts except the knees are locked to place the focus on the hamstrings.

#2 Standard Sets

- Barbell squats-6x6-15

- Hack squats-4x8-12
- Barbell leg lunges-3x10-12
- Leg extensions-4x12
- Toe presses on leg press-3x15
- Seated calf raises-3x12

Barbell squats are great for building overall mass in the upper legs. In fact, they stimulate muscle growth over the entire body due to their ability to affect the central nervous system. Therefore, to build new muscle on your arms one needs to be sure and train the legs hard or you will be shortchanging your arm training efforts.

Hack squats are best done on a hack squat machine because the machine eliminates the need to balance yourself and keeps you in the proper "groove" for the exercise. Leg lunges hit the leg muscles from a unique angle and are great for building thrust strength in them.

Seated calf raises and toe presses take all weight off the back, unlike standing calf raises which place heavy poundages on the spine.

#1 Superset
- Leg extensions-1x15
- supersetted with
- Hack squats-1x10
- Stair step-ups-1x12
- supersetted with
- Dumbbell squats-1x8
- Toe presses-1x15

- Seated calf raises-1x12

Initially do one complete cycle; more experienced bodybuilders can do an additional cycle after resting 2-3 minutes. Rest 1 minute between supersets.

Stair step-ups are done by holding a dumbbell in your left hand while stepping forward and up onto a step with your left leg. Squat down and push yourself up and back. After completing the desired amount of reps, switch to your right leg and hold the weight with your right hand. Complete the reps in the same way.

#2 Superset
- Leg extensions-1x12-15
- supersetted with
- Leg curls-1x12-15
- Front squats-1x12-15
- supersetted with
- Leg presses-1x6-12
- Dumbbell squats-1x8-10
- supersetted with
- Dumbbell rear lunges-1x12
- Toe presses-1x15
- supersetted with
- Seated front calf raises-1x12

Front squats require you to balance yourself differently than regular squats. The weight used is considerably less and they hit your quads in a different way. After cleaning the weight to your shoulders you should place the bar high on your shoulders and wrap your arms around the bar. This alleviates the heavy strain that your wrists would be subjected to otherwise.

#1 Giant Set

- Leg extensions-1x15
- Dumbbell leg lunges-1x12
- Hack squats-1x8-10
- Sissy squats-1x15
- Front squats-1x10
- Leg curls-1x12
- Stiff-legged deadlifts-1x8
- Front cable kicks-1x15
- Standing calf raises-1x20
- Donkey calf raises-1x12

84

Front cable kicks are a great exercise to isolate the frontal thigh muscles (quads) and build a huge pump. Donkey calf raises were popularized in the film Pumping Iron. If you get a chance to watch the movie look for the footage of Arnold Schwarzenegger bent over with several guys on his back, his feet on a block of wood, pumping his calves up and down, building an intense burn in them.

#2 Giant Set

- Barbell squats-1x6-15
- Hack squats-1x8-12
- Leg press-feet high on the footplate-1x6-12
- Front squats-1x15
- Leg lunges-1x12

- Step-ups-1x10
- Leg extensions-1x12
- Glute-ham raise-1x12
- Front foot lifts-1x12
- Seated calf raises-1x15

Leg presses with the feet placed high on the footplate train the frontal thighs but focus much of the resistance on the hamstrings. Step-ups are done with a dumbbell in each hand. Stand in front of a staircase and step onto the 2nd or 3rd step with your left leg, bending down deep. Push yourself up and back. Switch legs and repeat.

The glute-ham raise is done as follows: Place your ankles between the ankle roller pads with your feet on the vertical platform and position your knees on the pad with your lower thighs against the large padded hump. Position the weight plate against your upper chest or behind your neck.

From an upright position, lower your body by straightening your knees until your body is horizontal. Continue to lower your torso by bending your hips until your body is upside down. Raise your torso by extending your hips until fully extended. Continue to raise your body by flexing your knees until your body is upright. Repeat.

Front foot lifts are done by placing a barbell plate on the top front of your feet while sitting on a bench. Raise the front of your feet up, pause one second, and let the weights back down.

Both giant sets should be done with one cycle initially.

Advanced bodybuilders can do a second cycle after a two minute rest.

Leg Routines of Top Bodybuilders

Tom Platz-Mr. Universe-"Quadzilla"

- Barbell squats-12x5-20
- Hack squats-3x20-30
- Leg extensions-8x10-30
- Lying leg curls-6x7-20
- Standing calf raises-4x10-15
- Seated calf raises-4x10-15
- Hack machine calf raises-4x10-15

Lee Haney-Mr. Olympia-multiple winner

- Squats-6x6-8
- Leg extensions-4x8-10
- Lying leg curls-5x8-10
- Lunges-3x12-15

Bertil Fox-Mr. Universe

- Squats-6x8-15
- Barbell hack squats-5x8-10
- supersetted with
- Leg extensions-5x8-10
- Lying leg curls-5x8-15

Chris Dickerson-Mr. Olympia

- Angled leg press-8x8-10
- Squats-5x8-10
- Leg extensions-6x8-10
- Lying leg curls-8x8-10

Frank Zane-Mr. Olympia-multiple winner

- Leg extensions-6x8-20
- Leg curls-6x8-20
- Squats or Nautilus lunges-5x10

Lou Ferrigno-Mr. Universe

- Front squats-6x10-15
- Hack squats-5x10-15
- Leg extensions-5x10-15
- Lying leg curls-6x10-15
- Lunges-4x10-15

Shoulders

Anatomy

The main muscle group of the shoulders are the deltoids. They move the upper arms by contracting in different directions and are divided into three heads, the anterior on the front, medial or middle and the posterior or rear. In addition to these there are other small muscles in the shoulder that aide in movement called the rotator cuff.

The rotator cuff is easily injured if impinged, so it is important to avoid any exercises or movements that put the shoulders in unnatural positions. The most dangerous one is behind neck presses; another is the back exercise behind neck pull-downs.

Shoulder Routines

#1 Straight Sets

- Dumbbell overhead press-5x6-12
- Front dumbbell raises-3x12
- Side dumbbell lateral raises-3x12

- Bent-over cable raises-3x12
- Upright dumbbell rows-3x10

This routine makes use of dumbbells for overhead presses due to the greater range of motion they provide. During all three of the raises use smooth motion throughout; while doing front and side raises don't lift the dumbbells any higher than shoulder height or you risk injury to your rotator cuff. The upright rows help build the trap muscles to fill in the tie-in for the shoulder/back region.

#2 Straight Sets
- Flat bench prone dumbbell side laterals-3x12
- One-arm cable front laterals-3x12
- Barbell overhead presses-6x6-12
- Seated reverse machine flyes-3x12

#1 Superset
- One-arm lying side dumbbell raises-3x12
- supersetted with
- Front barbell raises-3x12
- Machine overhead presses-5x6-10
- supersetted with
- Cable bent-over laterals-3x12

One-arm lying side dumbbell raises are a great way to isolate the deltoid muscle with an accent on the medial, or middle head. Because you are lying on a bench you will literally be forced to use good form throughout the exercise.

Front barbell raises are very similar to dumbbell front raises with the exception that you are unable to turn the wrists out at the top, something that I feel is beneficial to angling the weight properly for maximum contraction of the delt muscle. That being said, barbells are a nice alternative.

#2 Superset
- Single dumbbell front lateral raise-3x12
- supersetted with
- Seated machine laterals-3x10
- Upright rows-3x10-12
- supersetted with
- Dumbbell Arnold press-3x6-10

Upright rows may be done using a barbell or a set of dumbbells. Use strict form and raise the weight until it is even with your shoulders. This avoids injury to the rotator cuff and allows a maximum contraction at the top of the exercise.

The Arnold press is done with a pair of dumbbells. Hold them at shoulder height parallel with each other. Press them up, rotating them until your palms face forward. Pause one second then return.

#1 Giant Set
- Seated machines presses-1x6-10
- Dumbbell shoulder shrugs-1x6-8
- Seated dumbbell side lateral raises-1x10
- Cable one-handed front lateral raises-1x12
- Seated reverse pek dek flyes-1x10
- Dumbbell Arnold press-1x6-10
- Machine upright rows-1x10-12

89

Do one cycle initially; add a second cycle after a 2 minute rest when ready (3-6 months training experience)

#2 Giant Set
- Barbell cleans-1x6-8
- Dumbbell presses one-handed alternated-1x6-8
- Barbell upright rows-1x6-8
- Seated front dumbbell raises-alternated-1x10
- Seated dumbbell side lateral raises-1x10
- Bent over cable raises-1x10
- Seated reverse pek dek flyes-1x10
- Rotator cuff rotations-1x10 each direction

Barbell cleans are an excellent exercise to build overall strength and development in the entire shoulder girdle.   90 While all muscles in the shoulder area are active in this lift, the traps benefit greatly from this exercise. Rotator cuff rotations are done as follows: Hold a light dumbbell in each hand at shoulder height, arms locked straight out. Begin by making circular rotations approximately 6 inches in size. After 10 reps change direction and do 10 reverse circles.

Shoulder Routines of Champion Bodybuilders

Frank Zane-Mr. Olympia-multiple-winner

- Machine seated presses-5x6-15
- Dumbbell upright rows-5x8-15
- One-arm dumbbell side laterals-5x8-12
- Dumbbell Bent-over laterals-5-8-12

Lou Ferrigno-Mr. Universe

- Smith machine front presses-4x8-10
- One-arm cable side laterals-4x8-10
- Cable bent-over laterals-4x8-10
- Cable upright rows-4x8-10

Lee Haney-Mr. Olympia-multiple winner

- Seated barbell press behind neck-4x5-10
- Front barbell raises-4x6-10
- Dumbbell side lateral raises-5x8-10
- Dumbbell bent-over laterals-3x8-10
- Dumbbell shrugs-3x10-15

Boyer Coe-Mr. Universe

- One-arm cable side lateral raises-2x10
- Prone incline lateral raises-2x10
- Seated machine presses-4x8
- Dumbbell shrugs-2x15
- Barbell shrugs-4x10

Lee Labrada-Mr. Universe winner

- Dumbbell side lateral raises-3x10
- Seated barbell press behind neck-3x10
- Seated dumbbell bent-over laterals-3x10

Tom Platz-Mr. Universe winner

- Barbell upright rows-8x6-15
- barbell seated presses-8x6-15
- One-arm dumbbell side lateral raises-8x6-15
- One-arm cable side lateral raises-8x6-15

Ron Teufel-Mr. USA

- Nautilus rear delt laterals-4x8-10
- Seated barbell press behind neck-4x8-10
- Standing dumbbell presses-4x8-10
- Dumbbell side lateral raises-4x8-10
- Dumbbell shrugs-4x8-10
- Seated dumbbell bent-over lateral raises-3x10

Larry Scott-Mr. Olympia first winner

- Standing dumbbell presses-5x6
- Prone incline dumbbell lateral raises-5x6-8
- Cable bent-over lateral raises-5x6-8

(preceding three exercises are a giant set)

- One-arm dumbbell side lateral raises-5x8

Chris Dickerson-Mr. Olympia-multiple winner

- Seated barbell press behind neck-6x6-12
- Dumbbell side lateral raises-6x8-10
- Seated dumbbell presses-6x8
- Seated dumbbell bent-over lateral raises-6x12-15

- Barbell upright rows-4x10-12

Franco Columbu-Mr. Olympia multiple winner

- Seated dumbbell side lateral raises-4x10

- Dumbbell bent-over lateral raises-6x10

- seated barbell press behind neck-4x8

- Dumbbell alternate front raises-3x8

- One-arm cable side lateral raises-3x10

Triceps

Anatomy

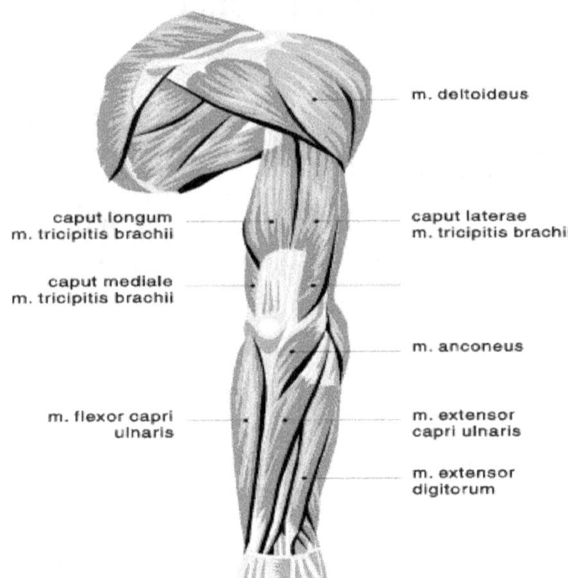

The triceps muscle contains three heads and originates at insertion points on the shoulder and elbow. It is responsible for straightening the arm from a bent position and pulling the upper arm forward and downward in a semi-circular motion. The tricep is fully-contracted when the arm is locked straight and the tricep is tensed hard. A great exercise to do this is the tricep kickback.

Bodybuilders looking to develop massive arms need to be aware that the tricep makes up 2/3 of total arm size. As much as bicep training is important, equally important is the development of the triceps. Every attempt must be made to develop the entire arm evenly or symmetry will be lost and injuries will result due to a strength imbalance.

The workouts contained in this section hit the triceps from all angles by using varying rep schemes (as with all muscle groups) and many of the almost infinite number of exercises available.

Most of the exercises in triceps training can be divided into overhead pressing, a form of bench press, downward pressing and rear pushing movements. We will be using all types for our training.

Triceps Routines

#1 Standard Sets

- Lying barbell triceps extension-4x10
- Seated one-dumbbell triceps extensions-4x12
- Standing cable triceps press-downs-4x6-10

- Seated machine tricep dips-4x6-10

An ez-curl bar may be used for the lying triceps extensions. Use a flat bench and bring the bar down to your forehead or behind your head to the bench. Seated machine triceps dips need to be done with the upper torso straight up to keep the tension on the triceps.

#2 Standard Sets

- Standing cable triceps power push-downs-4x6-12
- Seated machine triceps extensions-4x6-12
- High pulley forward angled triceps extensions-4x6-12
- Close-grip bench presses-4x6-12   95

Do the standing cable triceps power push-downs like regular triceps press-downs except point your elbows out to the sides and push straight down. This will build a strong, deep ache in your triceps.

#1 Superset

- Kneeling cable triceps extensions-3x6-10
- supersetted with
- Seated machine triceps dips-3x6-10
- Standing cable triceps kickbacks-3x10
- supersetted with
- Reverse-grip close-grip bench presses-3x8-10
- Seated inclined barbell extensions-3x8-10

- supersetted with
- Standing cable power push-downs-3x6-8

Do one cycle.

#2 Superset

- Cable power push-downs-4x10
- supersetted with
- Decline barbell triceps extensions-4x12
- One-dumbbell seated triceps extensions-3x10
- supersetted with
- Cable standing angled triceps extensions-3x8
- Reverse-grip bench press-3x8
- supersetted with
- Standing triceps dips-3x6-8

#1 Giant Set

- Reverse-grip bench press-1x6-8
- Seated machine triceps extensions-1x8-10
- Seated overhead cable triceps extensions-1x8-10
- Dumbbell triceps kickbacks-1x12
- One-arm cable push-downs-1x8-10
- Close-grip bench press-1x8
- Bench dips-1x10

Bench dips are done as follows: Place your hands on a bench approx. 24" apart while facing it with your backside. Place your feet up on a chair or 2nd bench in front of you. Lower yourself , pause and push yourself back up. Do one cycle initially; a second may be done by advanced trainees after a 3-4 minute rest.

#2 Giant Set
- Incline dumbbell tricep kickbacks-1x10
- Close-grip push-up-1x10
- Standing tricep dips-1x8-10
- Lying triceps extensions-1x10
- Incline cable triceps extensions-1x8
- One-arm cable push-downs palms-up grip-1x10
- Close-grip bench press-1x6-8

Do one cycle initially; a second may be done after a 3-4   97 minute rest- if an advanced bodybuilder.

Triceps Routines of Champion Bodybuilders

Sergio Oliva-Mr. Olympia winner

- Seated barbell triceps extensions-6x10-15

- One-arm dumbbell triceps extensions-6x10-15

- Cable push-downs-6x10-15

Larry Scott-Mr. Olympia winner

- Lying triceps extensions-6x6

- supersetted with

- Angled cable triceps extensions-6x6

- Kneeling cable triceps extensions-6x6

Lou Ferrigno-Mr. Universe winner

- lying triceps extensions with ez-curl bar-5x8-12
- Seated single-dumbbell triceps extensions-5x8-12
- Cable triceps push-downs-5x8-12

Robby Robinson-Mr. Universe winner

- Seated barbell triceps extensions-4x8-10
- Lying triceps extensions with ez-curl bar-4x8-10
- Cable triceps push-downs-4x8-10

Boyer Coe-Mr. Universe winner

- Cable triceps push-downs-4x8-10
- Lying triceps extensions with ez-curl bar-4x8-10   98
- One-arm dumbbell triceps extensions-4x8-10
- One-arm dumbbell triceps kickbacks-4x8-10

Chris Dickerson-Mr. Olympia winner

- Cable triceps push-downs-4x8
- Seated barbell triceps extensions-4x8
- Standing high-pulley,long cable triceps extensions-4x10
- Kneeling cable triceps push-downs-3x10

Mike Mentzer-Mr. Universe winner

- Cable triceps push-downs-1x6-8
- supersetted with
- Standing triceps bar dips-1x6-8

- Lying barbell triceps extensions-1x6-8
- Nautilus triceps extensions-1x6-8

Jusup Wilkosz-Mr. Universe winner

- Cable triceps push-downs-5x10-12
- Triceps bar dips-5x10-12
- One-arm dumbbell triceps extensions5x10-12
- One-arm cable triceps push-downs-5x10-12

Biceps   99

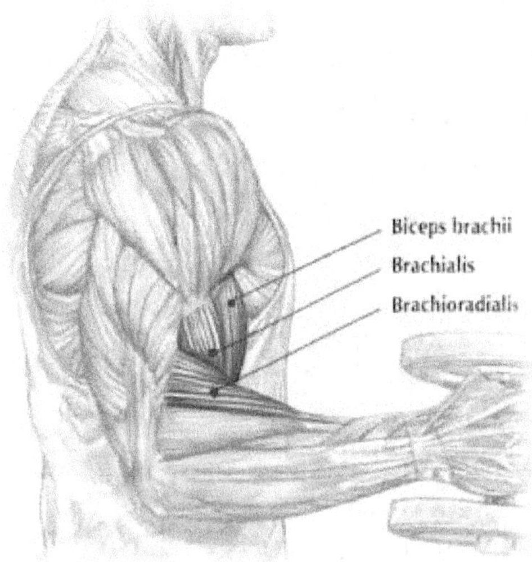

Anatomy

The biceps is a two-headed muscle that is located on the front of the upper arm and is responsible for flexing the forearm at the elbow and supinating it. The two heads, the long head and short head come together at an insertion point at the elbow.

The long head is located along the outer portion, while the short head is inside. Various exercises are used to focus on the different heads. Movements where the elbows are pulled back behind the body target the long head. Exercises that are done with the elbows in front of the body target the short head.

Grip placement and angle are altered in biceps exercises to target each head. To target the long head when using dumbbells or cables, the grip should be with the palms

102 facing each other.

If using a barbell the grip should be inside of shoulder width. To target the short head when using dumbbells or cables the grip should be supinated, where the palms are facing up.

Many beginning and advanced bodybuilders place an inordinate amount of training effort into building enormous biceps. Biceps have long been a symbol of strength and manhood-just ask anyone to "make a muscle" and they will invariably flex their arm in a biceps pose.

As stated in the section on triceps, the biceps account for only $1/3^{rd}$ of total arm size, so its important to remember to train your triceps as hard as biceps to build arms with great proportion as well as massive size.

One of the first well-known bodybuilders with great bicep development was John Grimek of York Barbell. He was both a bodybuilder and a weightlifter and excelled in both. Grimek won the Mr. America title in 1940-41 and used many exercises to work his biceps, sometimes doing one set of 8-12 different exercises.

Steve Reeves, who won the Mr. America title in 1947, had very well developed biceps due to his hard work and long muscle bellies. His upper arm measured nearly 19", which was very impressive especially for the time period.

Dumbbell incline curls were a favorite of Reeves, and were performed using very strict form. He felt they were an integral part of his biceps development.

Bill Pearl, a four-time Mr. Universe winner from the
103 1960's, had an upper arm girth of 20". He did a large
variety of exercises for his biceps and often topped out at 20
sets per workout.

No mention of bicep development would be complete
without mentioning Larry Scott, the first Mr. Olympia. Scott
used preacher curls so much while training biceps that the
exercise was affectionately renamed Scott Curls.

When looking to develop your biceps and assess your
potential, keep in mind that your ability to add mass to your
biceps, and your total arm size, is dependent on the length of
your muscle bellies. To check your potential for bicep size,
flex your arm in a single biceps pose and measure the
distance of the gap from your bicep to your elbow.

The larger the gap, the less potential you have for bicep
muscle mass. Don't get discouraged if your muscle belly is
shorter than average. Hard work and correct training will still
help you build impressive arm size.

Biceps Routines

#1 Standard Sets

- Barbell curls-4x6-10
- Seated incline dumbbell curls-3x8
- Dumbbell concentration curls-3x10
- Palms-facing cable pull-downs-2x8

Barbell curls should be done using strict form to keep the

pressure on the biceps and avoid injury. Seated incline
104 curls are great for hitting the biceps from a different
angle and keeping the resistance on the muscle.

Dumbbell concentration curls should be done sitting with
your hand placed on the knee on the same side as the arm
being trained. Place the elbow of the arm being trained on
your hand and curl the dumbbell up until the dumbbell
touches your shoulder. Flex the muscle hard before returning
the weight to the beginning position. Repeat.

#2 Standard Sets

- Machine curls-3x8-10
- Drag curls-2x8-12
- Preacher(Scott) curls-3x8-10
- Two-handed rope cable overhead curls-3x8-12

Curl machines tend to use a cam to vary the resistance placed
on the biceps, which allows you to train without hitting a
sticking point and keeps the weight on the muscle throughout
the exercise, something nearly impossible with standard
barbell curls.

#1 Superset

- Dumbbell concentration curls-2x8-10
- supersetted with
- Incline dumbbell curls-2x8-10
- Hammer curls-3x8
- supersetted with

- Barbell curls-3x6-8

Dumbbell concentration curls really "cramp" the muscle and activate a large number of muscle fibers if done properly. Tense the biceps hard at the top of the curl to increase the effectiveness of this.

Incline dumbbell curls eliminate the "dead zone" that is encountered in the barbell curl as a result of bad leverage angle. Since you will be using an incline bench it will be easier to have strict form. Tense the biceps hard at the top of the exercise.

Hammer curls target the Brachioradialis muscle which runs adjacent to the biceps muscle and ties into the forearm.

Barbell curls have a distinct disadvantage when it comes to leverage at the top of the lift. Because barbells offer linear resistance the force completely drops off at the top, allowing the muscle to rest. One way to counter this is to lean forward slightly so the resistance is maintained at the top of the curl. This slight change in angle completely changes the exercise, making it much more effective.

#2 Superset

- Machine curls-3x8-10
- supersetted with
- One-arm preacher curls-3x10 each arm
- Standing reverse curls-3x10-12
- supersetted with

- Close-grip chin-ups-3x8-10

Use a pair of dumbbells for the one-arm preacher curls.
Alternate by curling the left dumbbell first then the right one.
Standing reverse curls typically are used to train forearms but
build a nice tie-in between the bicep and forearm muscles.

Close-grip chins are the only compound exercise and use the
fresh lat (back) muscles to assist the biceps with the lift.

#1 Giant Set
- Lying flat bench curls-1x8-10
- Standing dumbbell curls-1x6-8
- Overhead cable rope curls-1x8-10
- Incline dumbbell curls-1x6-8
- Hammer curls-1x6-8
- Dumbbell concentration curl-1x10

The first exercise is to be done as follows: Lie face down on
a flat bench while holding a pair of dumbbells. Curl both up
as far as you can and tense your biceps hard for one second.
Repeat. Overhead rope curls are done with a double-rope
attachment which is affixed to the top pulley. With a neutral
grip, curl the rope handles down to the sides of your head.
Tense your biceps hard for one second before returning to the
top.

#2 Giant Set
- Barbell curls-1x8
- Dumbbell hammer curls-1x10
- Barbell drag curls-1x10
- Dumbbell preacher curls-1x12

- Mid-pulley one-arm rope curls-1x10
- Palms-facing chins-1x10

Barbell drag curls are done with a barbell beginning at the waist. With the bar against the body throughout, drag the bar up until its at the upper abs. Squeeze the biceps hard before returning. Mid-pulley one-arm rope curls are done as follows: Attach a one-hand rope pulley to the mid-pulley of a cable machine.

With a neutral grip, pull the handle toward your head until its at the side. Squeeze the biceps hard for one second before returning. Both giant sets consist of one cycle initially. A second can be done by advanced bodybuilders after a 2-3 minute rest.

Biceps Routines of Champion Bodybuilders

Lee Haney-Mr. Olympia-multiple winner

- Barbell curls-4x8-12

- Barbell preacher curls-3x8-12

- One-arm cable curls-3x10-15

Rich Gaspari-Mr. America winner

- Barbell curls-4x8-10

- Inclined dumbbell curls-3x8-10

- Barbell preacher curls-3x8-10

Sergio Oliva-Mr. Olympia multiple winner

- Barbell curls-6x8-10

- Seated alternate dumbbell curls-6x8-10
- Barbell preacher curls-6x8-10

Bertil Fox-Mr. Universe winner

- Barbell curls-4x8-10
- Barbell preacher curls-4x8-10
- Dumbbell incline curls-4x8-10
- Barbell concentration curls-4x8-10

The entire workout is done as a giant set. Go through all exercises with no rest. After completing one cycle, rest for two minutes then do a second giant set. Continue until all sets have been completed.

Frank Zane-Mr. Olympia-multiple winner

- Alternating dumbbell curls-4x8-10
- Cable preacher curls-4x8-10
- Low-incline dumbbell curls-4x8-10

Robby Robinson-Mr. Universe winner

- Barbell curls-4x8-10
- Incline dumbbell curls-3x8-10
- Standing dumbbell concentration curls-3x10-12

Gunnar Rosbo-European Amateur Champion

- Barbell curls-5x8-12
- Seated dumbbell curls-5x8-12
- Barbell preacher curls-5x8-12

- Seated dumbbell concentration curls-5x10-12   109

Lou Ferrigno-Mr. Universe winner

- Alternate dumbbell curls-5x8-10
- Incline dumbbell curls-5x8-10
- Close-grip barbell preacher curls-5x8-10
- Cable reverse curls-5x8-10

Chris Dickerson-Mr. Olympia-multiple winner

- Barbell curls-4x8-12
- Incline dumbbell curls-4x8-10
- Cable preacher curls-4x12
- Seated cable curls-4x10

Boyer Coe-Mr. Universe winner

- Barbell preacher curls-5x8-10
- Incline dumbbell curls-4x8-10
- Seated dumbbell concentration curls-4x8-10
- One-arm cable curls-4x8-10

Ed Corney-Mr. Universe winner

- Barbell curls-4x8-10
- One-arm dumbbell preacher curls-4x8-10
- Cable concentration curls-4x8-10

Larry Scott-Mr. Olympia multiple winner

- Incline dumbbell curls-3x6

- Dumbbell preacher curls-4x6
- tri-setted with
- Barbell preacher curls-4x6
- tri-setted with
- barbell reverse curls-4x6

Ron Teufel-Mr. USA winner

- Incline dumbbell curls-5x10
- One-arm cable curls-5x8-10
- Barbell curls-4x8-10

Arnold Schwarzenegger-Mr. Olympia-multiple winner

- Barbell curls-4x6-10
- Dumbbell curls-4x6-10
- Seated dumbbell concentration curls-4x6-10

Lee Labrada-Mr. Universe winner

- Barbell concentration curls-2x8-10
- Dumbbell preacher curls-2x8-10
- Alternating dumbbell hammer curls-2x8-10

Forearms

Anatomy

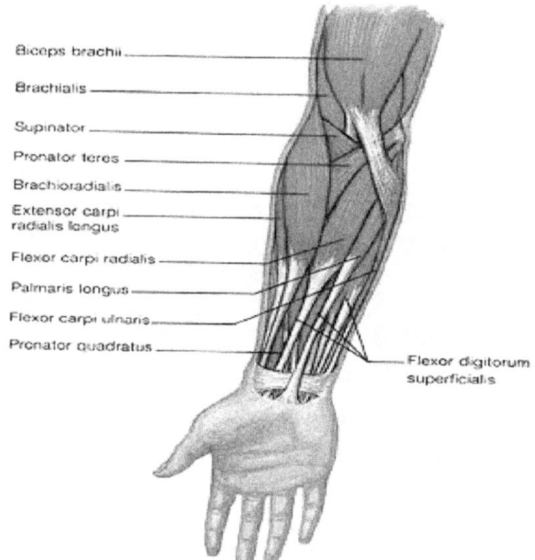

The forearms consist of the forearm supinator, flexor and extensors. The supinator is a large muscle located along the outside part of your forearm near your bicep and is responsible for exerting great force during such exercises as reverse curls and hammer curls.

The flexor muscles are a bundle of muscles located on the inside of your forearm and are involved during exercises that involve the flexing of your fist as in wrist curls.

The extensors are located on the outside of your forearm and extend your wrist upward as in reverse wrist curls. To develop your forearms completely it is necessary to train all three sections.

There is nothing that rounds out a great set of arms like a pair of massive forearms. Some bodybuilders never train their forearms directly-they get plenty of stimulation from

112

doing upper arm exercises and compound movements for chest, shoulders and back.

Others struggle to add an ounce of muscle on scrawny forearms and do countless sets of every exercise in the book. Done properly, routines to build strength and muscle size in the lower arms can be very effective.

Forearms Routines

Routine #1

- Barbell reverse curls-3x12-15
- Seated barbell wrist curls-3x15
- Seated barbell reverse wrist curls-3x15

Routine #2

- Dumbbell reverse preacher curls-3x12
- Standing barbell behind-the-back wrist curls-3x15
- Seated dumbbell reverse wrist curls-3x12

Both of these routines are a great way to build a strong burn in the forearms and stimulate them to grow. Do all three exercises with a short, one-minute rest between them.

Specialized Grip Building Routine

- Heavy hand grippers-3x15 squeezes
- Barbell pinch grip-3xone-minute pinch grip
- Claw grip-3x15 squeezes

Buy several sets of heavy hand grippers from a good gym supply house. Avoid the dept store brand as they wear out

quickly and don't provide a resistance heavy enough.
Squeeze the gripper until the handles touch on each rep.

To do the barbell plate pinch grip, pinch grip a barbell plate
and raise it off the floor, being careful to avoid dropping the
weight on your foot.

The claw grip is done with a special grip tool that is a sphere
made from durable rubber with many holes in it. Place your
thumb and fingers in the holes and squeeze the rubber pieces
together. This tool is great for performing squeezes at
different angles and gaps for complete development.

Forearm Routines of Champion Bodybuilders

Lee Haney-Mr. Olympia multiple winner

- Barbell reverse curls-5x6-10

- Barbell wrist curls-5x8-12

- Barbell reverse wrist curls-5x8-12

Larry Scott-1st Mr. Olympia winner

- Machine reverse curls-4x8

- seated barbell wrist curls-3x20

Dave Draper-Mr. Universe winner

- Barbell reverse curls-5x8-10

- Supported barbell wrist curls-5x5x10-15

Mike Christian-Grand Prix multiple winner

- Cable reverse curls-5x8-10

- Barbell wrist curls-5x10-12

- Barbell reverse wrist curls-5x10-12

Abdominals

Anatomy

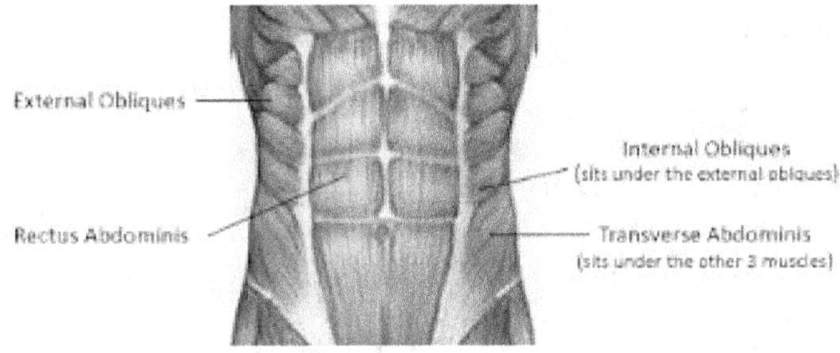

The ab region is made up of many different muscles. They include the rectus abdominus, the "six pack muscles in front of your stomach, external obliques, the muscles on the side that contract to twist your torso from side-side and intercostals, which aid in bending at the waist and pulling the torso front and to the side.

Ab Routines

Routine #1

- Roman chair sit-ups-3x15

- Hanging leg raises-3x20

- Machine crunches-3x15

- Dumbbell side bends-3x15 (each side)

Routine #2

- Floor crunches-4x15

- Leg raises-3x15

- Incline sit-ups-3x15

- cable side bends-3x20(each side)

Routine #3

- Machine crunches-4x20

- Leg raises on floor-3x20

- Roman chair sit-ups-4x15

- Machine rotary twists-3x25

Abdominal Routines of Champion Bodybuilders

Lee Haney-Mr. Olympia multiple winner

- Roman chair sit-ups-4x40-50

- Side bends-4x50-100

- Crunches-4x25-30

Tim Belknap-Mr. America

- Incline sit-ups-520-30

- Cable bench leg raises-5x20-30

- Side bends-5x30-50

Lou Ferrigno-Mr. Universe winner

- Roman chair sit-ups-4x50

- supersetted with

- Crunches-4x25

- Hanging leg raises-4x20

- supersetted with

- Cable crunches-4x30

Danny Padilla-Mr. Universe winner

- Roman chair sit-ups-4x25-50

- Seated twists-4x50-100

- Hanging leg raises-4x15-20

- Side bends-4x50-100

- Crunches-4x25-30

The entire routine is done as a giant set.

Ron Teufel-Mr. USA winner

- Incline sit-ups-2x100

- Roman chair sit-ups-2x100

- Flat leg raises-2x100

Alternate Training Routines

I have outlined straight set, superset and giant set routines for each muscle group. Now I'm going to give you additional training routines that will give you variety in your workouts to avoid boredom and be more productive developing the most muscle mass in the minimal time.

In previous sections we have discussed variations of the superset technique including antagonistic muscle supersets and the benefits of their use. One superset consisting of two exercises for the same muscle followed by two for the antagonistic muscle can be used or one exercise for the first muscle supersetted with an exercise for the antagonistic muscle works well, especially for chest-back and biceps-triceps.

Antagonistic Biceps-Triceps#1

- Barbell curls-4x6-10
- supersetted with
- Triceps push-downs-4x6-10
- Incline dumbbell curls-3x8-10
- supersetted with
- Lying triceps extensions-3x8-10

Antagonistic Biceps-Triceps#2

- Overhead rope cable curls-3x8-12
- supersetted with
- Seated overhead triceps extensions-3x8-12
- Palms-facing pull-downs-4x6-10
- supersetted with
- seated machine triceps dips-4x6-10

Antagonistic Chest-Back

- Pek flyes-3x10
- supersetted with
- Reverse pek flyes-3x10
- Incline machine bench press-6x6-10

- supersetted with
- barbell rows-6x6-10
- decline dumbbell bench press-4x6-10
- supersetted with
- Chin-ups-4x6-10

Antagonistic Legs-Quads-Hamstrings

- Leg extensions-4x12-15
- supersetted with
- Leg curls-4x12-15
- Barbell squats-8x4-12
- supersetted with
- Stiff-legged deadlifts-8x4-12

Antagonistic Abs-Lower Back

- Crunches-4x25
- supersetted with
- Roman chair hyper-extensions-4x20
- Good mornings-3x15
- supersetted with
- Incline sit-ups-3x25

Do these supersets the same way the others were done, resting 1-2 minutes between supersets.

Shocking Methods to Reinvigorate Growth

When a bodybuilder first begins weight training gains come quickly. The body is being subjected to overwhelming stress that hasn't been experienced before and reacts by quickly building new muscle mass to cope with it.

After awhile, despite training hard, both strength and size increases dwindle until frustration sets in and leads to a loss of interest in training.

The body has adapted to the training demands imposed on it and refuses to respond. The human body is very efficient and avoids using any more energy than it absolutely has to. Building muscle and maintaining it puts a huge burden on the body. It takes a lot of calories and nutrients to support large muscles and the body will do whatever it can to keep the status quo.

One way to restart growth and build new enthusiasm is to completely change the training regimen used, whether adding new exercises,changing rep counts, rest periods,etc. These will refresh your mind and subject your muscles to a completely new stimulus-leading to new growth.

Another way to break the sticking point barrier is to "shock" the muscles. You want to give them such an overwhelming stimulus that they can't do anything but respond. To do this we need to make our workouts radical. We'll add a lot of sets, increase the rep count drastically and/or add many more exercises. Frequency will be noticeably increased too.

The following routine is a great way to "shock" the legs. 120

- Barbell squats-10x10-100

- Leg press-12x15-100

- Leg extensions-10x25-100

- Leg curls-10x50-100

- Toe presses-10x50-100

As you can see, we have added many additional sets and reps, which necessitates reducing the weight from the loads that are typically used. This workout should build a strong burn in the muscle and will cause a powerful pump. Since it is so drastic, it will require a gradual increase in workload until you are able to complete the full routine unless you are already in great shape. Rest when needed and no more, keeping in mind that we are overtraining. This program needs to be short in duration or you will quickly breakdown the muscle and burn out.

Do this routine twice during one week then lay off leg work for one week resuming your normal program with one of the routines in this book.

This is a great routine to "shock" the biceps.

- Machine curls-10x15-100

- Concentration curls-10x50-100

- Palms-facing pull-downs-10x50-100

A great routine for "shocking" triceps:

- Seated dumbbell extensions-10x50-100

- Standing bar triceps dips-10x50-100

- Standing power triceps push-downs-10x50-100

Whole Body Training Routines

This system is old school and has the bodybuilder training the entire body during one workout. Split routines segment the body into different muscle groups which are trained on different days. Whole body routines use 2-6 sets total per muscle, which is a lot less than typical split routines. Since there are less sets than normal, recovery is faster so the muscles are able to be trained three times per week.

Three times per week training is a great way to boost the metabolism and burn extra body fat. It's also great for beginners because it allows them to condition their nervous system for more advanced training by getting them used to the various exercises used in bodybuilding making them more efficient at using the maximum amount of muscle fibers.

This form of training stimulates the release of testosterone and human growth hormone, two potent anabolic hormones, because of the leg, chest and back muscles being trained in the same workout. Science has shown that the more muscle mass being trained at one time, the more anabolic hormones are released.

The following is a routine for beginning bodybuilders:

- Barbell bench press-4x6-10
- Machine rows-4x6-10
- Seated machine lateral raise-3x10
- Leg press-4x8-15

- Incline dumbbell curls-3x8-10

- Lying triceps extensions-3x8-10

- Toe presses-3x15

- Machine crunches-3x20

For more advanced bodybuilders:

- Leg extensions-1x20

- Barbell squats-2x12-15

- Standing calf raises-2x20

- Incline dumbbell flyes-1x12

- Decline bench press-2x6-10

- Machine pullovers-1x12

- Barbell rows-2x6-8

- Dumbbell presses-2x6-10

- Cable curls-2x8-10

- Seated machine triceps extensions-2x8-10

- Crunches-2x25

Train three times per week with one of these whole body routines. Change the routines by substituting exercises with ones for the same muscle group.

Push-Pull Training 123

Push-pull training divides workouts into one session for pushing muscles and one for pulling muscles. The advantage is that muscles in the first workout are allowed to fully recover while the muscles in the second are trained. The arms are involved in all upper body training which often lead to overtraining so their training will be divided-biceps on pull days-triceps on push days.

Chest exercises involve triceps muscles as do many shoulder exercises. Back exercises involve biceps muscles. By dividing the body in this way the biceps are trained in the same session as the back and the triceps are trained in the same session as the chest and shoulders. This eliminates overuse of the arms and makes workouts more efficient. Train the pushing muscles first followed by two days rest then train the pulling muscles.

A great workout using this principle is:

Push

- Incline bench press-4x6-10
- Dumbbell presses-4x6-10
- Triceps kickbacks-3x10
- Leg press-6x8-15
- Standing calf raises-4x20

Pull

- Barbell rows-6x6-10
- Incline dumbbell curls-4x6-10

- Dumbbell shoulder shrugs-4x6-10

- Crunches-3x20

Push#2

- Barbell squats-6x8-12
- Standing bar dips-6x8-10
- Standing cable power push-downs-3x8-10
- Machine press-3x10

Pull#2

- Cable pull-downs-6x10
- Overhead cable curls-3x10
- Upright rows-3x8-10
- Leg raises-3x15

Most muscles are involved in pushing movements so your pull sessions will be much shorter than the pulling ones.

Feel free to substitute exercises for the same muscle group with others to add variety to your program.

Upper Body/Lower Body Split

Another effective way to divide your workouts is to separate them into upper and lower muscles. That way the upper body can be trained and allowed to recover while the lower body is trained and vice versa. Since the upper body involves more muscles it will be much more involved than the lower body.

On the other hand, the lower body involves the body's largest muscle mass so it will drain the body's resources more than the upper body does.

Upper Body

- Seated machine dips-3x8-10
- Incline bench press-4x8-10
- Decline dumbbell flyes-3x10
- Machine pullovers-4x10-12
- Machine rows-4x8-10
- Reverse machine flyes-3x10
- Roman chair hyper-extensions-3x12
- Dumbbell front raises-2x10
- Side lateral raises-2x10
- Dumbbell presses-3x8
- Barbell curls with bicep blaster-4x8
- Cable preacher curls-3x10
- Dumbbell triceps kickbacks-3x10
- Close-grip bench presses-3x10
- Hanging leg raises-2x15
- Machine crunches-2x20

Lower Body

- Leg presses-3x10-12
- Stair step-ups-3x10
- Standing leg curls-3x12
- Stiff-legged deadlifts-2x12

- Toe presses-2x15

- Seated calf raises-2x15

As in all medium-high volume training, use a weight that allows you to finish the desired rep count 1-2 reps short of muscular failure. If you were to end the sets at failure you would be unable to complete the required amount of sets and would have transitioned to high intensity training (HIT).

Pumping Routine

This technique begins with a compound exercise using low reps to build strength, adds a second compound exercise with moderate reps to build mass, uses an isolation movement with higher reps to build endurance and finishes with an isolation exercise using high reps to flood the muscle with blood to build a strong pump. This flushes away waste products, reduces muscle soreness in the days that follow and delivers nutrients and other building blocks to build muscle.

An example for the back is:

- Barbell rows-3x4-6

- Cable pull-downs-3x8-10

- Reverse pek dek-3x12-15

- Nautilus pullovers-3x18-25

Use a weight for each exercise that enables you to finish with the prescribed reps one rep before failure. All muscle groups large and small can benefit with this type of training.

Here is a routine for biceps:

- Palms-facing cable pull-downs-3x4-6
- Chins-3x8-10
- Incline dumbbell curls-3x12-15
- Concentration curls-3x20-25

And one for triceps:

- Close-grip bench press-3x4-6
- Seated machine triceps dips-3x8-10
- Triceps kickbacks-3x12-15
- Lying triceps extensions-3x20-25

And one for chest:

- Incline bench press-3x4-6
- Standing chest bar dips-3x8-10
- Cable crossovers-3x12-15
- Decline dumbbell flyes-20-25

100 Reps

This is a method of shocking a muscle into new growth because it introduces a rep scheme radically different than the one normally used. Whereas we normally do exercises using rep counts of 4-12, we are going to finish an exercise after completing one set of 100 reps.

The reps won't be completed in one shot but will involve doing a set of 70 reps to failure, putting the weight down to rest for 30 seconds and finishing the last 30 reps. This is a great way to build a powerful pump in the muscle as well.

An example of a routine for biceps is:

- Dumbbell preacher curls-1x100

Use dumbbells with a weight that leads to muscle failure at 70 reps (usually 20-25% of 1RM). Complete the reps, rest for 30 seconds, pick up a pair of dumbbells light enough to allow completion of 30 reps and finish with those.

This method is effective for all muscles. Remember to do one set of one exercise to failure twice as noted.

Multi-Angle

A great way to ensure that a muscle's fibers are receiving the necessary stimulation to grow to their fullest is to use multi-angle training. Not all fibers of a muscle are used in a given exercise and not all are trained effectively at certain rep counts. Multi-angle training insures all fibers in a muscle are recruited by using select exercises for each muscle.

Each of these exercises, while training the entire muscle, focus on different fibers within that muscle. Using the biceps as an example, barbell curls work the entire muscle but recruit certain fibers more than others. Concentration curls recruit yet another area, overhead cable curls yet another and so on.

A workout routine using this strategy will contain a large number of different exercises , with a low set count for each to keep the total muscle set count at an appropriate level.

Here are some routines for various muscle groups:

Legs

- Leg extensions-1x20
- Leg curls-1x20
- Forward dumbbell leg lunges-1x15
- Dumbbell step-ups-1x10
- Front barbell squats-1x10
- Leg press-1x8-10
- Standing calf raises-1x20
- Seated calf raises-1x15
- Barbell plate front raises-1x12

Legs

- Barbell squats-1x12
- Reverse dumbbell leg lunges-1x10
- Leg extensions-1x15
- Leg abductors-1x12
- Leg adductors-1x12
- Stiff-legged deadlifts-1x10
- Leg curls-1x15
- Donkey calf raises-1x15
- Standing calf raises-1x12

Chest

- Decline bench press-1x12

- Incline bench press-1x10
- Flat machine bench press-1x8
- Overhead Cable crossovers-1x15
- Incline dumbbell flyes-1x10
- Low pulley cable crossovers-1x10
- Seated machine chest dips-1x6-8
- Nautilus pullovers-1x12
- Decline dumbbell flyes-1x8

Chest

- Mid-pulley cable crossovers-1x10
- Push-ups-1x12
- High-pulley cable crossovers-1x12
- Incline machine bench press-1x8
- Decline machine bench press-1x6-8
- Standing bar dips-1x8
- Dumbbell pullovers-1x15
- Pek dek-1x10
- Chest compressions-1x8

Back

- Nautilus pullovers-1x12
- Machine rows-1x6
- Pull-ups-1x8-10

- Reverse pek flyes-1x10
- Lat pull-downs medium grip-1x10
- Low cable rows-1x8
- Dumbbell shoulder shrugs-1x8
- Dumbbell upright rows-1x10
- Machine lower back extensions-1x12

Back

- Barbell deadlifts-1x6
- Dumbbell rows-1x8
- Medium-grip palms-facing cable pull-downs-1x10
- Reverse pek flyes-1x10
- Dumbbell upright rows-1x12
- Mid-pulley cable rows-1x12
- End barbell rows-1x8
- High cable rows-1x8
- Roman chair hyper-extensions-1x12

Shoulders

- Front dumbbell raises-1x12
- Side dumbbell lateral raises-1x12
- Bent-over raises-1x12

- Machine presses-1x8

- Seated dumbbell alternate presses-1x10

- Rotator cuff dumbbell rotations-1x15

Shoulders

- Alternating dumbbell presses-1x6

- Cross-body angled cable raise-1x12

- Seated machine lateral raise-1x15

- Cable wood choppers-1x12 each side

- Inclined dumbbell presses-1x10

Biceps

- Concentration curls-1x12

- Preacher curls-1x10

- High cable curls-1x12

- Barbell curls-1x6-8

- Dumbbell hammer curls-1x8

- One-arm high cable curl-1x12

- Barbell reverse curl-1x6

Biceps   133

- Barbell curl-1x6

- Scott curl-1x8

- Incline dumbbell curl-1x10

- Dumbbell concentration curl-1x12

- Seated one-arm rope cable curl-1x10

- Dumbbell Zottman curl-1x8

- Barbell drag curl-1x6

Triceps

- Reverse-grip bench press-1x8

- Close-grip dumbbell bench press-1x10

- Seated dumbbell overhead tricep extensions-1x8

- Standing tricep cable push-downs-1x10

- Close-grip push-ups-1x10

- One-arm cable tricep kickbacks-1x12

Triceps

- One-arm dumbbell overhead tricep extensions-1x10

- Overhead cable tricep extension-1x12

- Decline dumbbell tricep extension-1x10

- Seated machine tricep dips-1x6

- Close-grip barbell bench press-1x8

- Reverse-grip one-arm cable tricep extension-1x12

Abs

- Incline bench sit-ups-1x20

- Machine crunches-1x20

- Incline bench leg raises-1x20

- Standing dumbbell side bends-1x20 each side

Each of these routines is ideal for training muscles from many different angles for the benefits discussed. Initially run through each routine once with a one minute rest between exercises. After using the routines for a couple of months, feel free to do a second cycle or a partial repeat of the routine, i.e. 1.5 routine (repeating half the exercises a second time). Train with moderate weights to allow completion of the desired rep count, ending the set at a difficulty level two reps before complete exhaustion of the muscle.

50-Rep Method

Use this technique to focus efforts on spurring new development on a lagging muscle. You will be training the chosen muscle with one exercise every day twice per day. Using chest as an example, do a set of bench presses either with a barbell, dumbbells or machine for 50 reps in the morning with a weight that causes mild fatigue in the muscle at the end of the set. Repeat 12 hours later with the same exercise and reps. Do this for 8 days straight then discontinue while reverting back to your former routine. You may do a different exercise every day to add variety.

Chest-1st day   135

- Dumbbell bench press-1x50-morning
- Dumbbell bench press-1x50-evening

2nd day

- Incline dumbbell flyes-1x50-morning
- Incline dumbbell flyes-1x50-evening

3rd day

- Cable crossovers high pulley-1x50-morning
- Cable crossovers-1x50-evening

4th day

- Decline barbell bench press-1x50-morning
- Decline bench press-1x50-evening

5th day

- Pek dek-1x50-morning
- Pek dek-1x50-evening

6th day

- Nautilus pullovers-150-morning
- Nautilus pullovers-1x50-evening

7th day

- Incline dumbbell bench press-1x50-morning
- Incline dumbbell bench press-1x50-evening

8th day

- Seated chest machine dips-1x50-morning
- Seated chest machine dips-1x50-evening

This is a program for chest with a good selection of daily

exercises and will bring good results by changing up the training you have been doing for chest, but is equally applicable for all other muscle groups. Select a good mix of isolation and compound exercises to thoroughly work the muscle from all angles.

One of the ways this works is by the building of new small blood vessels called capillaries, which help to increase the endurance and blood pumps in the muscle.

Unilateral Focus

Typically weight training involves the use of both limbs, or sides of the body, lifting,pressing or pulling a weight at the same time. While this is very effective if done properly, a great way to zero in on a lagging muscle is to train one side of the body at a time. In fact, each limb is stronger and able to exert more energy during an exercise than during a set using both limbs.

Some exercises that lend themselves to unilateral training are: cable curls, dumbbell curls, lat pull-downs, cable rows, dumbbell rows, leg press,leg extension, leg curl,tricep push-downs and dumbbell presses as well as many others.

The following routines are a great way to implement this training. After completing the first set with one arm or leg, switch to the other side and do the same.   137

Routine#1

Chest

- One-handed dumbbell flyes-1x12

- One-arm incline dumbbell flyes-1x12

- Incline one-arm bench press-1x8

- One-arm bench press-1x8

- One-arm machine dips-1x8

Back

- One-arm machine pullovers-1x15

- One-arm stiff-arm pull-downs-1x12

- One-arm dumbbell rows-1x8

- One-arm lat pull-downs-1x10

- One-arm Incline bench rows-1x6

Legs

- One-leg leg extensions-3x20

- supersetted with

- One-leg leg presses-3x12

- One-leg leg curls-3x20

- supersetted with

- One-leg stiff-legged deadlifts-3x15

- One-leg standing calf raises-2x25

- supersetted with

- One-leg toe presses-2x20

Shoulders

- One-hand dumbbell front lateral -3x15

- supersetted with
- One-hand dumbbell press-3x6-8

Biceps

- Seated dumbbell concentration curls-2x8
- supersetted with
- One-arm incline dumbbell curls-2x10
- One-arm dumbbell drag curls-2x8-10

Triceps

- One-arm cable overhead angle tricep extensions-2x10
- supersetted with
- One-arm cable tricep power push-downs-2x10
- One-arm dumbbell reverse bench press-2x6-8

Forearms

- One-arm dumbbell wrist curls-2x15
- One-arm dumbbell reverse wrist curls-2x15

Final Thoughts

This ends our medium volume training segment. While there are many additional techniques and strategies to effectively use this method of training, we have covered most of the 139 major ones in this book. Feel free to experiment with changing exercises, rep counts,etc to vary your training. This will accelerate your muscle gains and bring better results from your training.

HIT-High Intensity Training

This form of training stresses brief, less frequent workouts to build muscle and strength. It has extensive research backing up it's effectiveness even though the bodybuilding community has never fully embraced it. This is due to a number of reasons.

The bodybuilding establishment has always promoted their own form of training which utilizes a much lower intensity and a high set count which was designed around the desire to obtain a strong muscle pump. Set after set is done in an effort to rush blood into the muscle, leading to a tight, blood engorged condition.

While this is valuable due to the infusion of muscle-building nutrients and hydraulic pressure on the muscle cells, it isn't the most important factor in growing new muscle.

Study after study has shown that when a muscle is taxed sufficiently via resistance training small micro-tears result. The body takes these seriously enough to overcompensate by not only repairing the muscle but adding extra tissue as well. Over a period of time this growth becomes substantial enough to be measurable.

How does HIT differ from High Volume Training in its approach to building muscle? While High Volume Training uses many sets of sub-failure effort to work a muscle and pump it full of blood, HIT uses 1-3 exercises consisting of one set each per muscle training session.

All sets are taken to muscular failure , where it is impossible to crank out an additional rep. Many times HIT variables (see my book " DR HIT's Effective High Intensity Variables" for more information on HIT variables) are added to increase the intensity and take the muscle past the point of muscular failure.

Forced Reps

If we train using the barbell curl and wish to take the biceps to failure, we would load the bar with a heavy enough weight that causes us to finish the set at the point where we are unable to complete any additional reps. This constitutes the majority of sets in HIT Training.

But there is a necessity to go past this level of training to maximize the effectiveness of HIT. So instead of ending the set at the point of failure we have a training partner give us just enough assistance with lifting the bar to allow us to complete an additional 3-4 reps. This technique is called forced reps and is the most common of the HIT variables.

Forced reps are a great overloading technique and are very effective at conditioning muscles to use heavier weights. Make sure your training partner is giving just enough assistance to allow you to ring out extra reps otherwise you will miss out on the benefit of this technique.

If you normally go to failure during a set at 10 reps increase the weight so that you hit failure at 7 or 8 reps and have a partner assist you with completing another 2-4 reps.

Negative Reps

Studies have shown that the lowering portion of an exercise is the most effective at building strength. This is due to the ability of the bodybuilder to use weights that are 40% heavier while performing negative-only reps than is possible with traditional full reps.

There is a greater amount of micro-damage when doing negatives as well which can lead to greater muscle soreness two days after training so be cautious when initially using this technique.

So how do you do negative reps?

Using the incline bench press as an example, load the bar or machine with a weight that is 40% heavier than you normally use. Have two partners lift the bar by themselves until it is at the top of the press position.

Grab the bar while your partners slowly transfer the weight to you and lower the bar to your chest using an eight-count tempo. After the bar reaches your chest your partners lift the weight back up. Continue in this way until you are unable to safely control the descent of the weight.

This will bring a dull ache to your chest muscles due to the extreme intensity. Give negatives a try for all muscle groups.

What if you train alone and don't have the luxury of a training partner or two? Can you still do negatives? Yes. 142 For this we'll use Negative-Accentuated Reps. These are done in a similar fashion to negative reps with a slight twist.

Using the leg press as an example, push the footplate out to the pre-lockout position and pause one second before lowering the weight with your left leg only. Press the weight back out and lower with your right leg only.

Continue alternating between legs until you have hit failure. Because one leg is used to lower the weight there is more effective concentration of effort on the muscle, resulting in greater muscle in-roading.

Pre-Exhaust

Pre-exhaust was explained in the section on supersets so won't be elaborated on here. It is one of the most effective HIT techniques so make use of it often. Remember that there is absolutely no rest between exercises. As little as three seconds of rest allows 50% recuperation of the muscle, which defeats the purpose and effectiveness of this protocol.

Some examples of great pre-exhaust supersets are:

Legs

Leg extensions-1x15

Leg presses-1x10

Back

Nautilus pullovers*-1x15

Dumbbell Rows-1x8

*Other machines can be used or as an option dumbbell pullovers may be.

Chest

Incline dumbbell flyes-1x10

decline barbell bench press-1x8

Shoulders

Side deltoid raise machine-1x12

Standing barbell press-1x8

Biceps

Concentration curls-1x12

Seated machine rows palms-facing-1x8

Triceps

Standing overhead dumbbell triceps extensions -1x12

Bench dips-1x12

These are some workout routines using the pre-exhaust principle. More routines will be outlined in the chapters to follow.

Continuous Tension

One of the ways to activate a large number of muscle fibers is to keep the tension on the muscle throughout a set. A good way to do this is to avoid locking out on exercises like the leg press, bench press and triceps push-downs. Continuous tension goes one step further by making the movement during an exercise non-stop, thereby avoiding not only the lockout at the top of the exercise but any pause at the bottom of the exercise.

To compare traditional exercises to the continuous tension

version, do a set of dumbbell curls the normal way. After resting a couple of minutes, do the set again, but this time lean forward just enough to prevent the dead spot at the top of the curl. By leaning forward you keep the tension on the biceps at the top of the exercise and avoid any pause at the bottom.

After doing a set in this manner you will agree that it's necessary to reduce the weight below what you normally use in an exercise to compensate for the extra intensity generated with this type of training. Another benefit to this training is an intense pump in the muscle, which brings muscle-building nutrients into the muscle as well as an increase in hydraulic pressure in the muscle cells. This activates growth mechanisms in the muscle for new growth.

Zone (Partial) Reps

After you have been training for awhile you will invariably hit a sticking point in an exercise, where it is impossible to complete another rep. The bar or machine arm will stop at a certain point in the range of motion of an exercise.

Unfortunately, even though you are able to use a heavier weight in other portions of the rep you are limited in your progress by the sticking point. Zone, or partial reps were designed to bypass the sticking point, which allows each zone of the rep to be trained with the maximum weights possible to eliminate all sticking points.

To put this into practice let's take a look at the bench press. Typically, the sticking point in this lift is the point where the bar is at the ¾ mark-mere inches before lockout. This is the point where the smaller triceps take over much of the lifting from the stronger pectorals. The triceps are a much smaller muscle than the pectorals; this is where the weak link lies.

To use zone reps in the bench press we will divide the lift into three distinct zones, the bottom third, middle third and the top third. While free weight (barbells and dumbbells) are fine to use with this method, machines offer better control over movement and quicker weight changes.

Load the machine or barbell with a weight that allows 3-5 reps in the bottom zone and complete those reps to failure. Lower the weight 10% and do 3-5 reps in the middle zone. Reduce the weight another 10% and do 3-5 reps in the top zone.

After practicing this a few times it will be easy to target the maximum weights to use in each zone. Since there is no longer a sticking point, maximum weight can be used throughout the bench press, resulting in much improved gains in strength and size. The example presented is a common format but there are unlimited ways to apply zone reps.

For example, you could divide the bench press into two zones or four-five. You could train the top or middle zone first, change the weight, then train other zones to focus on other areas of the lift. Feel free to experiment with different combinations. This technique can be applied to almost every exercise in bodybuilding or powerlifting training with great success.

Power Rack Training

Heavy weights are necessary to build strength, power and muscle size. Certain exercises are dangerous when using heavy weights and training without a partner. The bench press is a great example. Who hasn't gotten stuck when repping out in the basement only to hit failure and feel the bar come back down on your chest? This can be extremely dangerous and could lead to a fatal outcome.

A common issue facing many bodybuilders is sticking points, as explained earlier. The weights keep piling on and lift totals keep going up and all of a sudden you hit a point where the gains come to a screeching halt and you are unable to eek out another rep. In the barbell squat this is the area between midway and the ¾ mark. This is the point where the leverage works against the legs, reducing the available strength output.

The best way to train through this is to do partial reps (see the section on zone partials) and the best tool to use is the power rack. This versatile tool comes to bodybuilding from the sport of powerlifting where it is used to train through sticking points and increase totals.

The power rack consists of two parallel uprights on each side . Pins are used as safety stops, racks and range-of-motion limiters. Using the bench press as an example, if we set the first set of pins at the beginning of the mid-point in the lift and the second pins at the upper-middle point, we can train the middle zone to the exclusion of the other zones.

Load a barbell with a weight that allows 6-8 reps to failure in the middle zone. Do one set of these, and on the last rep, push as hard as you can on the top pins for 10 seconds before returning the bar to the bottom pins.

Now train the upper zone, where the weak point is. Decrease the weight and set the pins at the bottom of the top zone. Set the second set of pins at the point prior to lockout. Press the bar for 6-8 reps and push hard at the top pin for 10 seconds before returning the bar to the pins.

This gives you a good idea how the power rack is used to train each zone of the bench press. The power rack gives you the ability to train each zone safely with different weights. The isometric 10-second push against the top pins increases the chest's strength and will result in heavier weights used during typical sets.

Power racks are great for training power exercises like squats, deadlifts and presses. The deadlift can be trained in different zones in much the same way the bench press was. The mid-point of the deadlift is the weak link. To build more strength in this zone set the bottom pins at the beginning of the middle zone and the top pins at the pre-lockout position.

Load the bar with a weight that allows 4-6 reps to failure. On the 6th rep, pull on the upper pin as hard as you can for 10 seconds before returning the bar to the bottom set of 148 pins. A full routine will be included in a later section.

Superslow

Ken Hutchins, an associate of Arthur Jones inventor of Nautilus Machines, devised a new style of training he called Superslow Training. It involves using a rep speed of 10 seconds for the concentric, or lifting phase and 4 seconds for the eccentric, or lowering phase.

Mr. Hutchin's reasoning for the slower seed was increased safety due to the absence of momentum and a more intense contraction in the muscle. He recommended use of Superslow training exclusively, avoiding the use of traditional training for the reasons above.

I agree that the slow rep speed eliminates momentum and reduces the chance of injury but disagree with his rejection of other forms of training. I value Superslow as a great addition to HIT training to be used in conjunction with the many other techniques available. Variety in training leads to better gains in the long run and proper high intensity training and exercise form have proven to be very safe with only a slight chance of injury.

Extended Slow Reps

A variation of Superslow, extended slow reps use a rep cadence of 30 seconds for the positive and 30 seconds for the negative. The very slow speed increases the intensity to a very high degree, therefore a set includes only one full rep.

The key issue is determining the correct amount of weight to use for the initial workout. Because of the intense nature of this method there will be an initial trial and error until the correct poundage can be determined.

I like to switch things up and do the positive portion first and other times do the negative in the beginning. Most exercises may be used with this protocol, some work better with the negative-first approach and others with positive-first.

Burn Reps

Burn reps allow the bodybuilder to extend a set past the point of positive failure by adding a series of short, pulsing type partial reps to the end of the set. These reps are appropriately named as you will see after trying them for the first time.

They cause an intense burn which results from the buildup of lactic acid in the muscle. The restriction of blood flow that results from this training causes an intense pump in the muscle.

Even though they are usually done at the end of a set they can be used effectively at the beginning and even in the middle of a set.

A barbell curl is a great exercise to illustrate this technique. Curl the bar until failure is reached. Do a series of 6-inch, rapid partial reps until you are unable to move the bar. As an alternative, curl the bar for four full reps then do a series of six burn reps in the middle zone before finishing the set with four full reps.

Occlusion 150

Japanese exercise researchers theorized if a pump leads to greater muscle mass due to both hydraulic pressure and the influx of nutrients in the muscle, increasing the pump might lead to even better results. KAATSU training was the result of their studies and was found to be both safe and effective. How does this newer style of training compare to traditional HIT training?

Conventional training uses moderate-heavy weights (80-90% of 1RM) for 6-12 reps to stimulate growth in muscles. Occlusion training restricts blood flow in the veins but not the arteries to increase the amount of blood in the muscle and decrease the flow out through the veins.

Due to the decreased oxygen level in the muscle, the slow-twitch fibers, which need oxygen to function and are called on first before fast twitch fibers during a typical set, are bypassed by the body in favor of fast twitch fibers to do the work. This leads to increased hypertrophy, or muscle size, because fast twitch fibers are the ones that are responsible for almost all muscle size increases.

So how do we safely restrict the blood flow? Most bodybuilders use resistance bands, blood pressure cuffs, wrist straps or cinch straps used for cargo hauling. The cuff should be placed at the joint just above the muscle being trained. If training arms put the cuff at the place just under the shoulder above the biceps or at the armpit.

If training legs, put the cuff at the very top of the leg below the hip. How tight should the cuff be? On a tightness scale of 1-10 the cuff should be a 5. For legs, the cuff should be slightly tighter. Keep the cuff on for the entire set and rest periods and remove it immediately after completing training, which should be more brief than your normal sessions.

Occlusion training gives the same or better results using only 20-50% of the weight used during standard sets of the same exercise. Complete no more than three sets for large muscles and two for smaller ones, such as arms and shoulders.

Rest-Pause

One of the problems bodybuilders face when training is ending a set due to lactic acid buildup instead of muscle fatigue. This is due to the extremely uncomfortable feeling lactic acid causes.

Rest-pause provides a great solution to this problem as well as allowing the muscle time to replenish phosphocreatine, which is used by muscles to produce greater strength output. Rest-Pause is done by lifting a weight that is at or near your maximum for one rep followed by a 10-second rest period then another rep and so on.

It will become necessary to reduce the weight after the second or third rep and continue to do so as the set progresses to allow the completion of full reps.

A workout for chest is as follows:

- Bench press-1x 8 (single max reps)

Set up the machine or barbell with 90% of your 1RM(1 rep max). Complete one rep, rest 10 seconds then repeat. Reduce the weight by 10-15% and do another rep. Continue until 8 reps have been completed.

- Seated machine dips-1x8 (single max reps)

Do these in the same manner as above. All reps should be max effort reps to gain the most growth benefit. There will be additional routines in the

Rest-Pause Alternatives

The rest-pause outlined in the above section is the traditional method used by HIT bodybuilders for years and has proved itself to be one of the most effective at producing new muscle growth and strength.

There are several other very good variations on this concept that are equally effective and allow you to use rest-pause while introducing variation in your training.

Three-Rep Method

In the original method we used a series of one-rep singles interspersed with 10-second rest periods. The three rep method allows the use of slightly lighter weights. It increases the total number of reps during the set which is good for increasing the Sarcoplasmic Fluid between the muscle's fibers. Since it involves a series of short, three-rep phases, it allows flushing of lactic acid similar to the traditional rest-pause.

The following is an example of a three-rep rest-pause workout for back:

- Barbell rows-1x6-3-rep bursts

Load the bar with a weight that is 85% of your 1RM. Using a smooth motion row the bar to your upper abdomen. Return the weight to the beginning position and repeat for a total of three reps. Set the bar down and rest for 10 seconds then do another three-rep series. Continue in this way until six series have been completed.

- Cable pull-downs-1x6-3-rep bursts

After selecting a weight that is 85% of your 1RM complete these exactly as you did the barbell rows.

Alternating Rest-Pause

A variation of the three-rep method, this technique eliminates the 10-second rest period and substitutes it with alternating of each side of the body. This allows the one side to rest while the other is lifting the weight and facilitates the flushing of lactic acid. Since one arm or leg is being trained at a time, more concentration goes into the training of each side. This allows the use of a heavier weight by each side than would be possible in a two-arm exercise. Naturally the more weight used -the more overload and the more muscle!

An example of training the biceps is as follows:

- Machine curls-1x3(left arm)1x3(right arm) 1x3(left arm)1x3(left arm)1x3(left arm)1x3(right arm) 1x3(left arm)1x3(left arm)

Continue alternating in this fashion until you have hit failure at 12 total reps per side.

- Dumbbell preacher curls-1x3(left arm) 1x3(right arm) 1x3(left arm)1x3(left arm)1x3(left arm)1x3(right arm) 1x3(left arm)1x3(left arm)

154

Continue alternating in this fashion until you have hit failure at 12 total reps per side.

This training will really tax the biceps hard due to its ability to rapidly switch effort from one side to the other. As mentioned previously, this is great for flushing out lactic acid and building a big pump in the biceps.

There will be additional routines outlined in the chapters to follow.

Omni-Contraction

This technique is another way to emphasize the negative portion of a rep. During each rep the eccentric, or positive is done in the same way as a Rest-Pause rep, which is a one rep max using a weight that is 90-95% of your 1RM for the initial rep. After the first rep reduce the weight 10%. After resting for 10 seconds do the second rep and so on until a set of 8 total reps have been completed in this manner. The negative part is done as follows: As the bar or machine handle is lowered it is stopped and held for 2-3 seconds one third of the way down, at mid-point and at the final third position.

The dumbbell bench press is done as follows:

Lower the dumbbells down to the chest, making sure to get a great stretch. Press the weight up to the pre-lockout position. Lower the weight one third of the way and hold for 2-3 seconds. Lower to mid-point and hold it for another 2-3 seconds. Lower it the weight to the bottom third and hold it for a final 2-3 seconds. Omni-contraction adds the benefit of static holds to a rest-pause set.

Infitonic

This form of training is similar to Rest-Pause and Omni-contraction training. Infitonic is done like Rest-Pause with a maximum positive, or concentric portion but the negative portion is increased to maximum exertion by having your training partner push down on the bar or weight to increase the resistance or load while you lower the bar. This increases the intensity of each rep over Rest-Pause levels.

An example of an Infitonic set of incline bench presses looks like this:

- Incline bench press-1x8

Load the barbell with a weight that is 90-95% of your 1RM and complete the positive. At the top your training partner places his/her hand on the bar and pushes down, allowing you to control the downward movement of the bar with maximum exertion. Rest 10 seconds, reduce the weight 10% and do a second rep in the same way and so on until a total of 8 reps have been completed.

Rolling Static Partials

This is a technique I developed and is a combination of several different protocols, including burn reps, static holds and partial reps. It's a great way to integrate the benefits 156 of each and offers the bodybuilder an intuitive method to further his/her muscle gains. I recommend bodybuilders waiting until they reach the advanced level of training before progressing to this technique.

To define this HIT variable I will use the barbell curl:

Begin the curl with a moderate weight. Curl the weight four reps, and at the beginning of the 5th rep, do a series of 4 burn reps followed by a 10-second hold. Continue doing reps by dividing the full rep into thirds. Do several partial reps in the middle zone of the curl before doing a series of several burn reps. Continue by doing several reps in the lower zone and finishing with a final 10-second hold. Reduce the weight by 15% and do a second set of 6 reps in the same way.

The key is to randomly do a series of burn reps, static holds and partial reps to "confuse" your body to reinvigorate growth. Experiment with different zones and holds.

Static Holds

With high intensity training it is imperative that one trains with the most effort possible. The goal should be to train with 100% effort, which is technically impossible but should be strived for nonetheless. One of the ways available to increase the intensity of your training is Static Holds.

These, like Rest-pause, have many different variations available. There are standard 10-second holds with no rest, 5-second rest and 10-second rest periods.

The idea is to load the bar or machine with a weight that is barely possible to hold for the required time period, be it 10 or 20 seconds. After each successive hold it will be necessary for a weight reduction of 10-15% to allow the next hold to take place.

Heavy weights carefully handled by training partners are a necessity. The best tools to use with static holds are selectorized strength machines because of their ease of use, ability to change weight quickly and their safety.

Initially, compound exercises were used exclusively but later isolation exercises showed their merit and they were added to training sessions.

Is There A Need To Use Full Range Of Motion In Exercises?

Many trainers will tell you that to properly train a muscle you need to go through an exercise's full range of motion. This is not completely true. Certain bodybuilders and powerlifters need to go through the full range of motion on an exercise or their strength will increase in the trained zone and lag in the zones that weren't trained.

Other trainees develop a full spectrum of strength by doing partial reps in limited zones. Therefore I recommend you train with a combination of full range of motion reps and zone partials, burn reps and static holds.

Partial reps are great for eliminating sticking points in an exercise. For instance, in the barbell row the lifter typically hits a sticking point where the bar stops moving three quarters through the lift.

This is due to the weaker biceps muscles taking over much of the pulling from the stronger back muscles. Unfortunately the weight used in the barbell row, or any other lift for that matter,is limited to the amount of weight that can be used throughout the entire lift.

To work the weak link in the barbell row, use a power rack if one is available. If one isn't available use a pair of dumbbells or a barbell. Set the lower pins on the power rack at the lower end of the sticking point and the top pins at the top.

Load the barbell with a weight that leads to failure at 8 reps. Pull the bar until it contacts the top pins and pull against the pins as hard as you can for five seconds before lowering the bar to the bottom pins. Keep repeating in this way until 8 reps have been completed to failure.

This is an example of the proper use of a power rack. I'll outline more training programs using this valuable free weight tool in a different chapter.

The point I'm making is to be flexible with your training and use all valid, scientifically proven techniques in your workouts to experience the best gains.

Static holds use no range of motion as they are just that-static holds. The benefit they provide is the result of a high recruitment of muscle fibers due to the force necessary to hold heavy weights motionless. Since there is very little movement, there is little buildup of lactic acid; any that does accumulate is removed by the body during the brief rest periods between holds. 159

The Different Static Hold Training Routines

The original way static holds were done is by loading a barbell or machine with a very heavy weight that can barely be held in position for 5-10 seconds before the weight begins to descend. The weight is reduced 10% while the bodybuilder rests for 10 seconds then the weight is held in position for another 10 seconds. This is repeated until 8 holds have been completed.

This is great for overloading the muscles and instigating a large amount of muscle fiber recruitment to complete the hold. It requires a very heavy weight to be used which has some drawbacks, the main one being an increased risk of injury and the necessity of training with assistants to help with lifting the incredibly heavy weights that are required.

A training program for chest using this protocol looks like this:

- Incline bench press with machine-1x8 max single holds interspersed with 10-second rest periods

An incline bench press machine is the best equipment to use for this training due to safety and ease of use. The first hold should be with a weight that is much heavier than you normally use in a standard incline bench press single attempt(1 rep max). Have your training partner(s) lift the machine's arm for you.

The hold position should be at the pre-lockout point. Hold the machine arm for 10 seconds, at which point it should begin lowering as your muscle strength fails. Lower it back down and rest for 10 seconds as your assistant reduces the weight 10%. Repeat for a second hold. Reduce the weight by another 10% and do a third hold. Continue until a total of 8 holds have been completed.

A training program for back using this protocol looks like this:

Machine rows-1x8 max single holds with a 10-second rest period in between holds

Do these in the same fashion as you did the incline bench press. With this training I can't emphasize enough the importance in putting forth 100% effort otherwise you will fail to push the muscles hard enough to recruit the maximum amount of muscle fibers. This is a sampling of a couple of workout routines. More will be outlined in the following chapters.

Pyramid Static Holds

Since the traditional method of training with static holds necessitates the use of extremely heavy weights and one or two training partners, an alternative was created which mimics the pyramid style of training prevalent in powerlifting.

Powerlifters begin by lifting a weight that is 50% of their 1RM for 3-5 reps then continue to work their way up in weight and down in reps until they max out in weight with 1-2 reps. They finish the lift by working their way back down in weight and increasing the reps.

161

With pyramid holds we begin by using a weight that is moderately heavy- one that can be comfortably held for 10 seconds. After a 10-second rest, the weight is increased and the weight is held for 10 seconds. Continue increasing the weight until a max weight is reached that can barely be held for 10 seconds.

Work your way back down the stack in the same way you worked yourself up. This allows you to quickly work your way up in intensity while preparing your muscles to handle heavier weights.

A workout for biceps looks like this:

- Incline machine curls-1x12 static holds

1st hold -50% of max 10-second hold, 2nd hold-60% of max 10-second hold, 3rd hold-70% of max 10-second hold, 4th hold-80% of max 10-second hold, 5th hold-90% of max 10-second hold, 6th hold-100% of max 10-second hold, 7th hold-90% of max 10-second hold, 8th hold-80% of max 10-second hold, 9th hold-70% of max 10-second hold, 10th hold-60% of max 10-second hold, 11th hold-50% of max 10-second hold, 12th hold-40% of max 10-second hold

Don't rest more than five seconds between holds. We want to tighten up the rest periods a little more than usual because we aren't hitting failure in the initial holds, unlike traditional max holds. The five second rest allows enough time for your body to flush the lactic acid from your muscles, preventing excessive burning and pain, two things that are guaranteed to end a set prematurely.   162

As you experiment with different max hold programs, you will find each gives your muscles a different stimulation. I find the standard holds really push my muscles, while the pyramid program gradually builds in intensity and brings about a strong, deep ache in the muscle.

Both are great ways to build muscle so I recommend you cycle between them to keep your workouts fresh and productive. Always strive to add weight to the machine every workout to overload the muscles and produce new growth and strength.

There is an additional form of static holds-one which uses extremely heavy weights with holds as little as 1/4-1 second!

This technique was developed by John Little, a personal friend of HIT pioneer, Mike Mentzer. John felt if static holds with heavy weights and hold times of 6-10 seconds were intense, holds with a duration of 1/4-1 second using even heavier weights would be more effective in building strength and size. He altered his method due to the heavier weights and shorter hold time as follows:

Chest

- Machine decline bench press -max weight, 1/4-1 second hold in contracted position x 4 holds

Have your training assistants lift the machine arms into the fully-contracted position and transfer the weight to you. Hold the weight motionless for 1/4-1 second. As the weight begins to descend, your partners quickly lift the arms back up.   163 Repeat this for three more holds then lower the weight back to the stack.

Back

- Machine rows-max weight, 1/4-1 second hold in contracted position x 4 holds

Perform these in the same manner as the decline bench press. With this exercise your partners pull the machine arms in toward you to the fully-contracted position.

Each muscle should be trained with maximum weights using compound exercises (see list later in this book).

With this form of static holds you get the benefit of maximum contractions due to the use of extremely heavy weights. The added strength that is derived from this training translates into larger muscles after the initial buildup of strength.

There is a greater possibility of injury if this isn't done properly due to the use of extremely heavy weights. As long as you have two experienced partners and stress the importance of a smooth transition of the weight you should be fine.

John Little feels that since the strong contractions realized through this method contribute to rapid muscle strength increase, training with repetitions is no longer needed. I feel it is necessary to train using a varied schedule of different HIT techniques and rep counts to stimulate all fiber types in a muscle and experience maximum growth in a muscle.   164

Isometric Training

Isometrics are similar to static holds in that there is no movement during a set and muscular force is exerted against a heavy or immovable object. With static holds the heavy object is a barbell or a machine's arms. In isometrics the immovable object is either the opposing muscle or an object that is fixed and unable to move. It could also be a barbell or machine's arms.

Isometrics eliminate much of the force from the muscle's tendons and ligaments and focus all effort on increasing the amount of fibers recruited in a muscle. The contractions during an isometric set are more intense than is possible with standard free weight and machine training.

This is a result of the activation of more motor units in the muscle than is possible with weight training. During an intense isometric contraction nearly all of the muscle's fibers are called into play. Strength gains of 14-40% were obtained over a 10-week period using isometric action training.

It's easy to focus the efforts on certain zones of an exercise to train past sticking points, or weak zones. During the barbell bench press, the bar moves off the chest as a result of the strong pectoral muscles. Around the mid-point, the deltoids and triceps take over , resulting in less force being generated due to these smaller, weaker muscles doing most of the pressing of the weight.

To train around this mid-zone weak link, set the pins in a power rack at the beginning of the middle zone. Use an 165 unloaded bar and press it into the pins attempting to push through the pins as hard as you can for 30 seconds before releasing the bar. Repeat this for a second rep after resting for one minute. Continue for a total of four reps during the initial workout. After a couple of weeks increase the rep count to six, never going beyond six total reps.

After training in this way you will feel a deep ache in your pecs due to the extreme contractions generated.

To train the deltoids, stand sideways next to a wall or other sturdy structure. Raise your arm up to the side about 3 inches until it contacts the wall and press as hard as you can, as if you are going to move the wall out of your way to allow you to raise your arm in a side delt raise.

Continue for 30 seconds before releasing your arm. Rest for 30 seconds before repeating for a second rep. Do a total of 4 reps initially, working up to six after a couple of weeks like you did in the bench press.

As with static holds and zone partials, train all zones of an exercise to train all zones evenly though it has been demonstrated isometrics develop strength in the entire range of motion of an exercise even if training is done only in one zone. This is especially true if the isometric was done in the weakest zone of a lift.

There are two ways to train using isometrics- the type just outlined-timed and stops.

Stops are done after reaching failure in a typical set. Chin-ups are a great example. After failing on your last rep -instead of ending the set-do a series of 5 second stops at four different locations on the way down.

Experiment with the different routines outlined further in this book including the ones combining isometric reps with conventional sets in a superset.

Sarcoplasmic Fluid

One of the factors in a bodybuilder's muscle size is the development of the Sarcoplasmic fluid. This is the fluid that surrounds a muscle's fibers and is increased with training using a moderately high time under tension or rep count.

I practice variation in my workouts to keep things fresh, the body guessing and the muscles growing. One session do static holds, the next use zone partials to break through sticking points, and another rest-pause or some other technique. With the current lineup of HIT variables the combinations are endless! More routines will be outlined in the following chapters.

HIT Training Routines

Pre-exhaust

Legs

- Leg extensions-1x15
- supersetted with no rest
- Leg press-1x12
- Dumbbell leg lunges-1x12 each side

Legs#2

- Leg extensions-1x20

- supersetted with no rest
- Barbell squat-1x10
- Dumbbell leg step-ups-1x10 each side

Legs#3

- Leg extensions-1x15
- supersetted with no rest
- Leg lunges with dumbbells-1x12 each leg
- Standing leg curls-1x12

Chest

- Pek flyes-1x12
- supersetted with no rest
- Incline dumbbell bench press-1x6-8
- Standing bar dips-1x6

Chest#2

- Decline dumbbell flyes-1x12
- supersetted with no rest
- Seated chest machine dips-1x8
- Mid-pulley cable crossovers-1x10

Chest#3

- High-pulley cable crossovers-1x15
- supersetted with no rest
- Flat barbell bench press-1x6

- Nautilus pullovers-1x10

Back

- Nautilus pullovers-1x12
- supersetted with no rest
- Machine rows-1x8
- Reverse pek dek flyes-1x12

Back#2

- Stiff-arm lat pull-downs-1x10
- supersetted with no rest
- Seated medium-grip, palms-facing pull-downs-1x6-8
- High cable rows-1x10

Back#3

- Reverse pek dek flyes-1x12
- supersetted with no rest
- Palms-facing pull-ups-1x10
- Barbell dead-lift-1x8

Shoulders

- Seated machine lateral raise-1x12
- supersetted with no rest
- Machine press-1x8

Shoulders#2

- Dumbbell front raises-1x12

- supersetted with no rest
- Dumbbell alternate presses-1x6-8

Shoulders#3

- Cable cross-body lateral raise-1x12
- supersetted with no rest
- Smith machine barbell presses-1x6

Biceps

- Cable curl-1x10
- supersetted with no rest
- Seated palms-facing cable pull-downs-1x8

Biceps#2

- Incline bench dumbbell curls-1x10
- supersetted with no rest
- Palms-facing bent over barbell row-1x8

Biceps#3

- Dumbbell Zercher curls-1x10
- supersetted with no rest
- Chin-ups-1x8

Triceps

- Standing angled high-pulley cable tricep cable extensions-1x8
- supersetted with no rest

- Dumbbell narrow bench press-1x10

Triceps#2

- seated single-dumbbell tricep extensions-1x10
- supersetted with no rest
- Standing bar tricep dips-1x6-8

Triceps#3

- Seated cable power push-downs-1x12
- supersetted with no rest
- Close-grip push-ups-1x10

Note: There aren't any direct compound exercises for forearms and abs so I recommend doing a regular routine for those muscles.

Abs

- Stomach crunches-1x25
- supersetted with no rest
- Leg raises-1x25

Forearms

- Reverse barbell curls-1x10
- Barbell wrist curls-1x25

Double Pre-Exhaust 171

Legs

- Leg extension-1x15
- supersetted with no rest
- leg adductor-1x15
- supersetted with no rest
- Barbell squats-1x10

Legs#2

- Leg extensions-1x20
- supersetted with no rest
- Leg curls-1x20
- supersetted with no rest
- front barbell squats-1x12

Chest

- Decline dumbbell flyes-1x10
- supersetted with no rest
- Incline dumbbell flyes-1x10
- supersetted with no rest
- flat dumbbell bench press-1x6-8

Chest#2

- High-pulley cable crossovers-1x12
- supersetted with no rest
- Low-pulley cable crossovers-1x12
- supersetted with no rest

- Standing bar dips-1x8

Chest#3

- Pek dek flyes-1x10
- supersetted with no rest
- Nautilus pullovers-1x10
- supersetted with no rest
- Seated chest dips-1x8

Back

- Stiff-arm lat pull-downs-1x10
- supersetted with no rest
- Seated reverse pek dek flyes-1x10
- supersetted with no rest
- Chin-ups-1x10

Back#2

- Nautilus pullovers-1x12
- supersetted with no rest
- Ab strap pull-downs-1x8
- supersetted with no rest
- Seated machine rows-1x6

Back#3

- Reverse pek dek flyes-1x12

- supersetted with no rest
- Stiff-arm lat pull-downs-1x10
- supersetted with no rest
- Deadlifts-1x6

Shoulders

- Front lateral raises-1x12
- supersetted with no rest
- Bent-over raises-1x12
- supersetted with no rest
- Barbell presses-1x8

Shoulders#2

- Rotator cuff dumbbell rotations-1x15 each direction
- supersetted with no rest
- Incline dumbbell front raises-1x12
- supersetted with no rest
- Seated cable presses-1x8

Shoulders#3

- Seated machine lateral raises-1x10
- supersetted with no rest
- Upright rows-1x8
- supersetted with no rest
- Standing barbell press-1x6

Biceps

- Concentration curls-1x12
- supersetted with no rest
- Barbell drag curls-1x10
- supersetted with no rest
- Palms-facing cable pull-downs-1x8

Biceps#2

- Lying dumbbell curls-1x10
- supersetted with no rest
- Lying cable curls-1x12
- Palms-forward barbell rows-1x8

Triceps

- Standing cable power push-downs-1x10
- supersetted with no rest
- Dumbbell triceps kickbacks-1x12
- supersetted with no rest
- Close-grip push-ups-1x10

Triceps#2

- Lying palms-down tricep extensions-1x10
- supersetted with no rest
- Standing bicep blaster one-handed tricep press-downs-1x10

- supersetted with no rest
- Bench dips-1x8

Forearms

- barbell wrist curls-1x15
- supersetted with no rest
- Barbell reverse wrist curls1x15
- supersetted with no rest
- Barbell reverse curls-1x8

Abs

- Ab machine crunches-1x20
- supersetted with no rest
- Hanging leg raises-1x15
- supersetted with no rest
- Ab wheel-1x10

Omni-Contraction

Note: Each rep has a negative with three 10-second static holds, one at the top,mid-point and near the bottom. See previous explanation for more detail.

Legs

- Leg extensions-1x15-normal execution
- Leg curls-1x15-normal execution
- Leg press-1x8-Omni-contraction

- Standing calf raises-1x20-normal execution

Legs#2

- Barbell squats-1x8-Omni-contraction
- Dumbbell leg lunges-1x12 each leg-normal execution
- Stiff-legged deadlift-1x10-normal execution
- Donkey calf raises-1x20-normal execution

Back

- Barbell row-1x8-Omni-contraction
- Medium-grip palms-facing pull-downs-1x12-normal execution
- Seated reverse pek dek flyes-1x10-normal execution
- Roman chair hyper-extensions-1x15-normal execution

Back#2

- Nautilus pullovers-1x12-normal execution
- End barbell row-1x6-normal execution
- Barbell deadlift-1x6-Omni-contraction
- Barbell good mornings-1x10-normal execution

Chest

- Pek dek flyes-1x12-normal execution
- Decline dumbbell flyes-1x10-normal execution
- Incline dumbbell bench press-1x8-Omni-contraction

Chest#2

- Barbell bench press-1x8-Omni-contraction
- Incline machine bench press-1x10-normal execution
- Low-pulley cable crossovers-1x12-normal execution

Shoulders

- Incline bench side lateral raises-1x10-normal execution
- Standing barbell press-1x8-Omni-contraction
- Dumbbell upright rows-1x10-normal execution

Shoulders#2

- Machine press-1x8-Omni-contraction
- One-arm cable cross-body lateral raises-1x10-normal execution
- Shoulder shrugs-1x8-Omni-contraction

Biceps

- One-hand rope hammer cable curl-1x8-Omni-contraction
- Overhead cable curl-1x12-normal execution

Biceps#2

- Cable concentration curl-1x10-normal execution
- Barbell drag curl-1x8-Omni-contraction

Triceps   178

- Seated cable overhead extension-1x10-normal execution

- Reverse-grip bench press-1x8-Omni-contraction

Triceps#2

- Standing cable triceps kickbacks-1x12-normal execution

- close-grip bench press-1x8-Omni-contraction

Forearms

- Windups-1x5-normal execution

- Reverse wrist curls-1x12-normal execution

Forearms#2

- Power squeezes-1x10-normal execution

- Reverse curls-1x8-Omni-contraction

Abs

- Incline sit-ups-1x20-normal execution

- Machine crunches-1x20-normal execution

Abs#2

- Lying leg raises-1x25-normal execution

- Reverse crunch-1x20-normal execution

Rest-Pause

Review the section on Rest-Pause Training before proceeding. All sets are to be done to failure.

Legs

- Leg press-1x8-Rest-pause

- Leg extensions-1x25-normal execution

- Leg curl-1x20-normal execution

- Standing calf raises-1x25-normal execution

Legs#2

- Leg lunges-1x12 each side-normal execution

- Leg step-ups-1x10 each side-normal execution

- Leg press-1x8-Rest-Pause

- Seated calf raises-1x20

Chest

- Seated machine dips-1x8-Rest-Pause

- Mid-pulley cable crossovers-1x12-normal execution

- Incline bench press-1x10-normal execution

Chest#2

- Incline dumbbell flyes-1x10-normal execution

- Decline dumbbell bench press-1x8-normal execution

- Flat machine bench press-1x8-Rest-Pause

Back

- Seated machine rows-1x8-Rest-Pause

- Deadlift-1x6-normal execution

- Seated reverse pek flyes-1x12-normal execution

- Good mornings-1x15-normal execution

Back#2

- Nautilus pullover-1x12-normal execution
- High rows-1x10-normal execution
- Deadlift-1x8-Rest-Pause

Shoulders

- Machine presses-1x8-Rest-Pause
- Incline dumbbell front delt raise-1x10-normal execution

Shoulders#2

- Seated machine delt raises-1x12-normal execution
- Machine presses-1x8-Rest-Pause

Biceps

- Barbell drag curl-1x8-Rest-Pause
- Barbell Scott Curl-1x10-normal execution

Biceps#2

- Lying dumbbell curls-1x12-normal execution
- Standing barbell curl-1x8-Rest-Pause

Triceps

- Seated tricep machine dips-1x8-Rest-Pause
- Seated ez-curl tricep extensions-1x12-normal

execution

Triceps#2

- Standing cable tricep kickbacks-1x10-normal execution

- Reverse-grip barbell bench press-1x8-Rest-Pause

Do one of the previous routines for abs and forearms as they are not well suited for Rest-Pause training.

Alternate Rest-Pause

Refer to the section on the alternate rest-pause technique before attempting these routines.

Legs

- Leg press-1x3x6 (a total of 6, 3 rep sequences with 10 second rest breaks in-between)

- Front barbell squats-1x15 (standard set)

- Leg extensions-1x20 (standard set)

- Lying leg curl-1x20

- Donkey calf raises-1x20

Chest

- Barbell bench press-1x3x6 (a total of 6, 3 rep sequences with 10 second rest breaks in-between)

- Incline dumbbell bench press-1x6 (standard set)

- Decline dumbbell flyes-1x10 (standard set)

Back

- Barbell rows-1x3x6 (a total of 6, 3 rep sequences with 10 second rest breaks in-between)

- Pull-ups-1x10 (standard set)

- Nautilus pullovers-1x12 (standard set)

- Machine back extensions-1x15 (standard set)

Shoulders

- Machine presses- 1x3x6 (a total of 6, 3 rep sequences with 10 second rest breaks in-between)

- Two-handed cable lateral raises-1x12 (standard set)

Biceps

- Machine curls-1x3x6 (a total of 6, 3 rep sequences with 10 second rest breaks in-between)

- Barbell drag curls-1x8 (standard set)

Triceps

- Bar dips 1x3x6 (a total of 6, 3 rep sequences with 10 second rest breaks in-between)

- Seated machine tricep extensions-1x8 (standard set)

Forearms

- Reverse curls-1x3x6 (a total of 6, 3 rep sequences with 10 second rest breaks in-between)

- Barbell wrist curls-1x20 (standard set)

Abs

- Machine crunches 1x3x6 (a total of 6, 3 rep

sequences with 10 second rest breaks in-between)

- Hanging leg raises-1x20 (standard set)

Forced repetitions

Legs

- Leg press-1x12+3 forced reps (use arms to assist legs with forced reps)

- Front squats-1x12 (no forced reps)

- Leg extensions-1x20+2 forced reps (partner-assisted)

- Toe presses on Leg press machine(no forced reps)

Back

- Nautilus pullovers-1x10+4 forced reps (partner-assisted)

- Machine rows-1x6-8 (no forced reps)

- Palms-facing cable lat pull-downs-1x10+3 forced reps (partner-assisted)

- Barbell good mornings-1x15

Chest

- Pek dek flyes-1x10+4 forced reps (partner-assisted)

- Incline dumbbell bench press-1x10 (no forced reps)

- Seated machine dips-1x6+3 forced reps (partner-assisted)

Shoulders   184

- Seated machine lateral raises-1x8+3 forced reps (partner-assisted)

- Standing barbell presses-1x6-8 (no forced reps)

Biceps

- Preacher curls-1x8+3 forced reps (partner-assisted)

- Overhead one-handed cable curls alternated-1x8+ 3 forced reps each arm (use free hand to assist with forced reps)

Triceps

- One-handed cable tricep kickbacks-1x8+3 forced reps (partner-assisted)

- Reverse-grip bench press-1x8+3 forced reps (partner-assisted)

Forearms

- Reverse barbell curls-1x8+3 forced reps (partner-assisted)

- Gripper squeezes-1x15 each hand (no forced reps)

Abs

- Lying ab crunches-1x25 (no forced reps)

- Machine leg raises-1x20 (no forced reps)

Continuous Tension

Refer to the section on continuous tension training for more information before proceeding with the following routines.

Legs

- Leg extensions-1x20 (Extend your legs to the top and flex hard. Lower the machine arms down, stopping at the bottom making sure to keep your leg muscles under tension at all times.)

- Leg press-1x15 (same as above. Avoid lockout at the top and keep tension on the leg muscles throughout.)

- Lying leg curls-1x15 (Keep tension on the hamstrings.)

- Standing calf raises-1x15 (Keep tension on the calf muscles throughout. This will build a very strong burn in your calves.

Back

- V-handle cable pull-downs-1x10 (Keep tension on by limiting the range of motion to the beginning stretch at the top and squeeze hard when the handle reaches your chest.)

- Machine rows-1x8 (Keep the tension on the back muscles throughout the set.)

- Cable high rows-1x10 (Row a double handle to the upper chest area. Squeeze hard at the full contraction point.)

- Roman chair hyper-extensions-1x15 (Bend down low at the beginning and bring yourself up until your torso is above parallel.)

Chest

- Pek dek flyes-1x12 (Get a good stretch at the beginning and keep tension on the pecs. Don't bring the machine's arms together to avoid reducing the tension on the pecs.

- Low-pulley cable crossovers-1x10 (Bring the handles upward at an angle, keeping tension on the pecs.)

- Seated machine dips-1x6 (Lean forward to accent the chest. Avoid lockout and resting at the top of the exercise.)

Shoulders

- Seated machine lateral raise-1x12 Keep the tension on the delts by limiting the range of motion at the bottom.

- Upright row with dumbbells-1x10 Limit the range of motion to one that keeps tension on the shoulders. In other words, avoid going to the bottom and don't raise the weight above shoulder level.

Biceps

- Machine curls-1x10 Machine curls make it easy to keep resistance on the biceps. Get a good stretch at the bottom and build to a strong contraction at the top.

- Rope hammer curls-1x8 Attach a rope to both low pulleys on a crossover machine. Curl the weights up to a strong contraction and avoid going to the bottom of the curl to keep resistance on the muscles.

187

Triceps

- Standing cable push-downs-1x12 Don't let the handle come up too high to keep the resistance on the triceps.
- Triceps kickback with dumbbells-1x12 Don't bring the dumbbells too far forward to avoid taking the resistance off the muscles.

Abs

- Hanging leg raises-1x25 Keep the legs from going to the bottom to keep resistance on the abs.
- Roman chair sit-ups-1x25 Use a range of motion that allows the muscle to experience resistance throughout the exercise.

Forearms

- Grip squeezes-1x25 Use heavy grippers with a full range of motion, keeping the resistance on the forearms.
- Reverse barbell curls-1x8 Keep tension on the muscles at all time.

Standard Static Holds

Chest

- Machine bench press-1x8 (10-second holds with a 10-second rest in-between) (Reduce the weight 10% after each hold to facilitate completion of the next hold.)
- Pek dek flyes-1x4 (10-second holds with a 188 10-second rest in-between) (Reduce the weight 10% after each hold to facilitate completion of the next

hold.)

Back

- End barbell row-1x8 (10-second holds with a 10-second rest in-between) (Reduce the weight 10% after each hold to facilitate completion of the next hold.)
- Reverse pek dek flyes-1x4 (10-second holds with a 10-second rest in-between) (Reduce the weight 10% after each hold to facilitate completion of the next hold.)

Legs

- Leg press-1x8 (10-second holds with a 10-second rest in-between) (Reduce the weight 10% after each hold to facilitate completion of the next hold.)
- Leg extensions-1x4 (10-second holds with a 10-second rest in-between) (Reduce the weight 10% after each hold to facilitate completion of the next hold.)
- Standing calf raises-1x8 (10-second holds with a 10-second rest in-between) (Reduce the weight 10% after each hold to facilitate completion of the next hold.)

Shoulders

- Machine presses-1x8 (10-second holds with a 10-second rest in-between) (Reduce the weight 10% after each hold to facilitate completion of the next hold.)

Biceps

- Machine preacher curls-1x8 (10-second holds with a 10-second rest in-between) (Reduce the weight 10%

after each hold to facilitate completion of the next hold.)

Triceps

- Standing cable triceps power push-downs-1x8 (10-second holds with a 10-second rest in-between) (Reduce the weight 10% after each hold to facilitate completion of the next hold.)

Forearms

- Seated barbell wrist curls-1x8 (10-second holds with a 10-second rest in-between) (Reduce the weight 10% after each hold to facilitate completion of the next hold.)

Abs

- Seated machine crunches-1x8 (10-second holds with a 10-second rest in-between) (Reduce the weight 10% after each hold to facilitate completion of the next hold.)

Note: Smaller muscles like biceps, triceps and shoulders, which are also involved in back and chest training, are trained with one set of 8 holds while larger muscles like legs, chest and back, have a second exercise with one set of 4 holds, which is 1.5x's the workload of the smaller muscles.

Pyramid Static Holds 190

Chest

- Incline bench press-1x6 up and 6 down (Select a weight that is 80% of your max 10-second hold weight. Hold the weight for 10-seconds at the full contraction point just prior to lockout, rest for 10 seconds before repeating with a weight that is 10% heavier than the first. Continue working up the stack until you max out with a weight that you can barely hold for 10 seconds. Work back down the stack as you reduce the weight for each hold.)

Back

- Barbell rows-1x6 up and 6 down (Select a weight that is 80% of your max 10-second hold weight. Hold the weight for 10-seconds at the point of max contraction at the upper abs, rest for 10 seconds before repeating with a weight that is 10% heavier than the first. Continue working up the stack until you max out with a weight that you can barely hold for 10 seconds. Work back down the stack as you reduce the weight for each hold.)

Legs

- Leg press- 1x6 up and 6 down (Select a weight that is 80% of your max 10-second hold weight. Hold the weight for 10-seconds at the point of max contraction near lockout, rest for 10 seconds before repeating with a weight that is 10% heavier than the first. Continue working up the stack until you max out with a weight that you can barely hold for 10 seconds. Work back down the stack as you reduce the weight for each hold.)

Shoulders

- Seated machine press-1x6 up and 6 down (Select a weight that is 80% of your max 10-second hold weight. Hold the weight for 10-seconds at the point of max contraction near lockout, rest for 10 seconds before repeating with a weight that is 10% heavier than the first. Continue working up the stack until you max out with a weight that you can barely hold for 10 seconds. Work back down the stack as you reduce the weight for each hold.)

Biceps

- Dumbbell preacher curl-1x6 up and 6 down (Select a weight that is 80% of your max 10-second hold weight. Hold the weight for 10-seconds at the point of max contraction near the top, rest for 10 seconds before repeating with a weight that is 10% heavier than the first. Continue working up the stack until you max out with a weight that you can barely hold for 10 seconds. Work back down the dumbbell rack as you reduce the weight for each hold.)

Triceps

- Lying dumbbell tricep extensions-1x6 up and 6 down (Select a weight that is 80% of your max 10-second hold weight. Hold the weight for 10-seconds at the 192 point of max contraction near lockout, rest for 10 seconds before repeating with a weight that is 10% heavier than the first. Continue working up the dumbbell rack until you max out with a weight that you can barely hold for 10 seconds. Work back down the rack as you reduce the weight for each hold.)

Forearms

- Reverse barbell wrist curl-1x6 up and 6 down (Select a weight that is 80% of your max 10-second hold weight. Hold the weight for 10-seconds at the point of max contraction at the top, rest for 10 seconds before repeating with a weight that is 10% heavier than the first. Continue working up the rack until you max out with a weight that you can barely hold for 10 seconds. Work back down the rack as you reduce the weight for each hold.)

Abs

- Ab machine crunches-1x6 up and 6 down (Select a weight that is 80% of your max 10-second hold weight. Hold the weight for 10-seconds at the point of max contraction, rest for 10 seconds before repeating with a weight that is 10% heavier than the first. Continue working up the stack until you max out with a weight that you can barely hold for 10 seconds. Work back down the stack as you reduce the weight for each hold.)

It will take a couple of workouts to perfect the amount of weight used for the first hold and amount the

weight needs to be reduced for each successive hold, but a 10% reduction is ideal in most cases.

Pyramid static holds reduce the amount of weight needed by beginning with a sub-maximum load and quickly building up to a max weight before reducing weight on each successive hold. This gives an appropriate stimulus to the muscle while greatly reducing the chance of injury.

One set of one exercise is used for each muscle due to the level of intensity. Resist the common temptation to add sets and exercises or you will quickly overtrain.

Pure Negative

Chest

- Machine bench press-1x8

Load the machine with a weight that is 40% more than you use during normal sets. Have a partner(s) lift the weight with their strength exclusively. After they transfer the weight to you lower it to a count of 8. Repeat for a total of 8 negatives, which should be the point where you are no longer able to safely control the downward movement of the machine's arms.

- Pek dek flyes-1x6 Load the machine with a weight that is 40% more than you typically use. These are done in the same way the machine bench presses were. The machine arms should be pressed together until they touch by your partner. Resist the machine's   194 arms opening to a count of 8. Repeat for a total of 6 reps.

Back

- Cable pull-downs-1x8 Select a weight 40% higher than normal. Have your partner pull the bar to your chest and transfer the weight to you. Resist the descent of the weight to a count of 8. Do a total of 8 negatives.

- Reverse pek dek flyes-1x6 Do these in a similar fashion as the pek dek flyes except reverse them to work the upper back.

Legs

- Leg press-1x8 Select a weight 140% higher than normal. Two partners will be needed to lift the footplate into the fully-extended position. Resist the footplate to a count of 8. An alternative would be to help in the extension of the footplate by pressing on your legs with your arms.

- Leg extensions-1x6 Use a weight 140% of your normal weight. After the extension arms are lifted into position, lower them to a count of 8.

Shoulders

- Machine presses-1x8 Same method as previous exercises, 140% of normal weight, partner lifts the machine arms into position at the top, resist them to a count of 8.

- Cable lateral raise-1x4 Use a weight 140% of normal load. Have your partner lift the handles into a shoulder height position and lower to a count of 8. Repeat.

Triceps

- Machine reverse bench press-1x8 Same method as previous exercises, 140% of normal weight, partner lifts the machine arms into position at the top, resist them to a count of 8.

- Seated single-dumbbell overhead tricep extensions-1x4 Have your partner lift the dumbbell to the point prior to lockout. Lower the dumbbell slowly to a count of 8.

Forearms

- Reverse wind-ups-1x8 Use a small bar with a rope and clip on the end. Attach a barbell plate to the end of the rope. Have a partner wind the rope around the bar and hand it to you. Holding the bar at waist height, unwind the rope and lower the weight to the floor. Repeat for a total of 8 cycles. Note: Since the forearms get a lot of work with all upper body training they need one set to break them down sufficiently.

Abs

- Machine ab crunches-1x8 Select a weight that is 140% of the weight you use for standard machine crunches. Have your partner lift the machine's arm forward and transfer the weight to you. Resist the machine as you sit upright using an 8 count.

Peak Contraction

Legs

- Leg extensions-1x20 Extend your legs to the full contraction position and flex your thighs hard for 5 seconds. Do several burn reps and flex your thighs again. Repeat for a set of 20 reps.

- Step-ups-1x15 Use a pair of moderate weight dumbbells for this exercise. Stand in front of stairs and take a deep step up onto the second step and sink down deep. Push yourself up to just prior to lockout and do a series of burn reps before flexing your thigh hard. Repeat for a total of 15 reps for the left leg before training the right in the same way.

- Donkey calf raises-1x20 Use a donkey calf raise machine with a moderate weight selected. Press the weight up with your calves while keeping your knees locked. Flex your calves hard at the top for 5 seconds before lowering for a full stretch. Repeat for a total of 20 reps.

Chest

- Pek dek flyes-1x15 Bring the arms of the machine toward each other, stopping just before they touch and squeeze your pecs hard for 5 seconds. Do a series of burn reps, flex your pecs again before returning the weight to the stack. Repeat for a total of 15 reps.   197

- Decline machine bench press-1x10 Bring the

machine's arms down to get a full stretch before pressing them up, stopping just prior to lockout. Flex your pecs hard for 5 seconds then do a series of burn reps. Repeat.

Back

- Nautilus pullovers- 1x12 Bring the machine's arms to the end point and flex your lats hard for 5 seconds before doing a series of burn reps. Repeat for a total of 12 reps.

- Machine rows-1x8 Pull the handles toward you until they are parallel with your chest. Squeeze your back muscles hard for 5 seconds before doing a series of burn reps. Repeat for a total of 8 reps.

- Roman chair hyper-extensions-1x12 Use a weight plate to increase the resistance if needed. Lift yourself up until you are just above parallel and flex your lower back muscles for 5 seconds before doing a series of burn reps. Repeat for a total of 12 reps.

Shoulders

- Seated machine laterals-1x12 Bring the machine's arms up to parallel and flex your delts hard for 5 seconds before doing a series of burn reps. Repeat for 12 reps.

- Standing barbell press-1x8 Press the bar up to the pre-lockout position and flex your delts for 5 seconds   198 before doing a series of burn reps. Repeat for 8 reps.

Biceps

- Dumbbell preacher curls-1x12 Curl the dumbbells up to the top and flex your biceps for 5 seconds before doing several burn reps. Repeat for 12 reps.

- Incline dumbbell curls-1x8 Using an incline bench, curl the dumbbells up to the top, flex your biceps for 5 seconds and do several burn reps before repeating for a total of 8 reps.

Triceps

- Cable triceps kickbacks-one-arm-1x12 Pin your elbow to your side for this exercise. Push the handle back behind you and flex your tricep for 5 seconds before doing several burn reps. Repeat for a total of 12 reps before switching arms.

- Close grip dumbbell bench press-1x8 Hold the dumbbells approx. 18" apart. Press them up to the pre-lockout point and flex your triceps for 5 seconds before doing several burn reps. Repeat for 8 reps.

Forearms

- Leaning-forward reverse ez-curl reverse curls-1x10 Lean forward placing your forehead against a wall in front of you. Curls the bar up to the top and flex your forearm/biceps muscles for 5 seconds before doing a series of burn reps. Repeat for 10 reps.

Note that we are doing one set for forearms due to their heavy use during nearly all upper body training.

Abs

- Machine crunches-1x25 Curl forward all the way and flex your abs for 5 seconds before doing a series of burn reps. Repeat for 25 reps.

We are doing one set due to the risk of overtraining abs since they are a small muscle.

Cheat Reps

Chest

- Barbell bench press-1x10 Load the barbell with a weight that is 110% of the weight you normally use in this lift. Use good form to complete as many reps as you can before bouncing the bar off your chest to help you press it up to the pre-lockout position.

- Seated machine chest dips- 1x10 Select a weight that is 110% of your normal weight. Complete as many reps as you can in good form before using momentum to assist in the completion of additional reps.

Back

- Barbell rows-1x8 Load the barbell with a weight that is 110% of your normal weight. Complete as many reps as you can in good form before using momentum to allow the completion of additional reps.

- Cable machine pull-downs 1x10 Use a weight that is 110% of your normal weight. Finish as many reps as you can in good form before using a slight jerking motion to aid in pulling the handle down to complete additional reps.

Shoulders

- Barbell press- 1x10 Load the barbell with 110% of your normal weight. Complete as many reps as you can in good form before using body momentum in the body to allow yourself to complete additional reps with the heavier weight.

- Standing dumbbell side lateral raises- 1x12 Use a weight 110% heavier than normal. Do as many reps in good form as you can before using a little body momentum to allow yourself to complete the additional reps.

Biceps

- Barbell curl- 1x10 Use a weight 110% of your normal weight. Do as many reps as you can in good form before using body momentum to assist yourself in completing additional reps.

- Palms-facing pull-downs- 1x10 Use a weight 110% of your typical weight. Complete as many reps as you can using good form before using a slight jerking motion to allow the completion of the final reps.

Triceps

- Overhead dumbbell triceps extensions- 1x12 Use a weight 110% of your usual weight. Complete as many reps as you can before using some momentum to allow yourself to complete the final reps.

- Close-grip barbell bench press – 1x8 Use a weight 110% of your normal weight. Complete as many reps as you can before using some momentum to allow yourself to complete additional reps.

Occlusion Training

Legs

- Barbell squats-1x12 Use a weight that is 30% of your typical weight. Attach a blood-flow restriction band around your upper thigh being careful not to over tighten. On a scale of 1-10, tighten the band to a 5.

- Leg extensions-1x15 Keep the band on while doing this exercise.

- Lying leg curl-1x15 Keep the band on while performing this exercise.

- Seated calf raises-1x25 Complete this exercise with the band on. Remove the band after finishing this exercise.

Chest

- Incline dumbbell flyes-1x12 Use a weight that is 30% of your typical weight. Place a blood-flow restriction band around the upper thigh of each leg and a band around both upper arms. On a scale of 1-10, the arm restriction should be a 3-4.

- Seated machine dips-1x8 Keep the bands on for this exercise. Remove the bands after finishing this exercise.

Back

- Lat pull-downs parallel grip-1x12 Use a weight that is 30% of your typical weight. Place a blood-flow restriction band around the upper thigh of each leg and a band around both upper arms. On a scale of 1-10 the arm restriction should be 3-4.

- High cable rows-1x8 Keep the bands on for this exercise.

- Lower back machine extensions-1x15 Keep the bands on for this exercise. Remove the bands after completing the set.

Shoulders

- Upright rows-1x12 Use a weight that is 30% of your typical weight. Place a blood-flow restriction band around both upper arms. On a scale of 1-10 the arm restriction should be 3-4.

- Incline dumbbell presses-1x8 Keep the bands on for this exercise. Remove the bands after finishing this exercise.

Triceps

- Standing cable power push-downs-1x10 Use a weight that is 30% of your typical weight. Place a blood-flow restriction band around both upper arms. On a scale of 1-10 the arm restriction should be 3-4.

- Single dumbbell overhead triceps extensions-1x8 Keep the bands on for this exercise. Remove the bands after finishing this exercise.

Biceps

- Overhead cable curls-1x10 Use a weight that is 30% of your typical weight. Place a blood-flow restriction band around both upper arms. On a scale of 1-10 the arm restriction should be 3-4.

- Cross-body dumbbell hammer curls-1x8 Keep the bands on for this exercise. Remove the bands after finishing this exercise.

Forearms

- Grip squeezes-1x25 Use a weight that is 30% of your typical weight. Place a blood-flow restriction band around both upper arms. On a scale of 1-10 the arm restriction should be 3-4.

Extended Slow Reps

Legs

- Leg press-1x1 (30 second positive-30 second negative)
- Leg extensions-1x25 (standard set)
- Standing calf raises-1x1 (30 second positive-30 second negative)

Back

- Machine rows-1x1 (30 second positive-30 second negative)

- Stiff-arm lat pull-downs-1x12 (standard set)
- Good mornings-1x20 (standard set)

Chest

- Machine bench press-1x1 (30 second positive-30 second negative)
- High pulley cable crossovers-1x12 (standard set)

Shoulders

- Machine presses-1x1 (30 second positive-30 second negative)
- Seated machine delt raises-1x12 (standard set)

Biceps

- Barbell drag curl-1x1 (30 second positive-30 second negative)
- Dumbbell preacher curl-1x10 (standard set)

Triceps

- Reverse barbell bench press-1x1 (30 second positive-30 second negative)
- Lying ez-curl triceps extensions-1x10 (standard set)

Forearms

- Reverse barbell curl-1x1 (30 second positive-30 second negative)

- Gripper squeezes-1x30 (standard set)

Abs

- Machine crunches-1x1 (30 second positive-30 second negative)
- Hanging leg raises-1x20 (standard set)

Pure Negative

Routine#1

Chest

- Decline machine bench press-1x8 (lower to a count of 8)
- Pek dek flyes-1x8 (lower to a count of 8)

Legs

- Leg press-1x8 (lower to a count of 8)
- Machine hack squat-1x8 (lower to a count of 8)
- Toe presses-1x8 (lower to a count of 8)

Back

- Machine rows-1x8 (lower to a count of 8)
- Nautilus pullovers-1x8 (lower to a count of 8)
- Machine back extensions-1x8 (lower to a count of 8)

Shoulders

- Machine presses-1x8 (lower to a count of 8)
- Side lateral raises-1x8 (lower to a count of 8)

Triceps

- Seated machine triceps extensions-1x8 (lower to a

count of 8)

- Machine dips-1x8 (lower to a count of 8)

Biceps

- Standing dumbbell curls-1x8 (lower to a count of 8)

- Palms-facing cable pull-downs-1x8 (lower to a count of 8)

Forearms

- Wind-ups-1x6 (lower to a count of 8)

Abs

- Machine crunches-1x8 (lower to a count of 8)

Routine#2

Legs

- Step-ups-1x8 (lower to a count of 8) Lower deep as usual but instead of pushing up step back and repeat the negative motion only.

- Leg extensions-1x8 (lower to a count of 8) Have your partner lift the machine's arm up and transfer the weight to you.

- One-legged dumbbell calf raises-1x8 (lower to a count of 8)

Chest

- Standing bar dips-1x8 (lower to a count of 8) Use a dip belt to add weight as needed to sufficiently overload your muscles.

- Machine bench press-1x8 (lower to a count of 8)

Back

- Lat pull-downs palms-facing-1x8 (lower to a count of 8)

- V-bar cable rows-1x8 (lower to a count of 8)

- Roman chair hyper-extensions-1x8 (lower to a count of 8) Use a weight plate held behind your head to overload your muscles.

Shoulders

- Cable front lateral raises-1x8 (lower to a count of 8)

- Bent-over lateral raises-1x8 (lower to a count of 8)

Biceps

- Machine curls-1x8 (lower to a count of 8)

- Chin-ups-1x8 (lower to a count of 8) Use a dip belt to add weight as needed to overload your biceps.

Triceps

- Single dumbbell overhead extensions-1x8 (lower to a count of 8)

- Barbell close-grip bench press-1x8 (lower to a count of 8)

Forearms

- Reverse dumbbell curls-1x8 (lower to a count of 8)

Abs

- Machine crunches-1x8 (lower to a count of 8)

Isometric Routines

Pure Isometric

Routine #1

Chest

- Barbell bench press-1x6-30-second iso-presses (2 at each of 3 zones)(Set pins on power rack so bar stops at the top of each zone)

- Chest squeezes-1x6-30-second iso-squeezes

Back

- Barbell rows in power rack-1x6-30-second iso-pulls (2 at each of 3 zones)(Set pins on power rack so bar stops at the top of each zone)

- Stiff-arm pull-downs-1x6-30-second iso-pulls (2 at each of 3 zones)(Have partner hold plates on stack to prevent movement during iso-pulls)

Legs

- Leg extensions-1x6-30-second iso-presses (2 at each of 3 zones)(Have partner stop and hold machine's arms at each zone)

- Leg presses against wall-1x6-30-second iso-presses (2 at each of 3 zones)(Hold firmly onto a stable seat and press hard against wall)

- Leg curls-1x6-30-second iso-pulls (2 at each of 3

zones)(Have partner stop and hold machine's arms at the top of all zones)

- Toe presses against wall-1x6-30-second iso-presses (2 at each of 3 zones)(1x6-30-second iso-presses (2 at each of 3 zones)

Shoulders

- Machine presses-1x6-30-second iso-presses (2 at each of 3 zones)(Have partner stop and hold machine's arms at the top of each zone)

Biceps

- Barbell preacher curls-1x6-30-second iso-curls (2 at each of 3 zones)(Have partner stop and hold barbell at the top of each zone)

Triceps

- Seated tricep extensions- 1x6-30-second iso-presses (2 at each of 3 zones)(Have partner stop and hold barbell at the top of each zone)

Abs

- Machine crunches- 1x6-30-second iso-crunches (2 at each of 3 zones)(Have partner stop and hold machine at the top of each zone)

Forearms

- Grip squeezes-1x6-30-second iso-squeezes (2 at each of 3 zones)(Squeeze hard statically at each zone)

Routine #2

Chest

- Pek dek-1x6-30-second iso-squeezes (2 at each of 3 zones)(Have partner stop and hold machine at the top of each zone)

- Machine bench presses-1x6-30-second iso-presses (2 at each of 3 zones)(Have partner stop and hold machine at the top of each zone)

Back

- Reverse machine flyes-1x6-30-second iso-flyes (2 at each of 3 zones)(Have partner stop and hold machine at the top of each zone)

- Pull-ups-1x6-30-second iso-pulls (2 at each of 3 zones)(Have partner stop and hold your body to prevent movement at the top of each zone)

Legs

- Leg extensions-1x6-30-second iso-presses (2 at each of 3 zones)(Have partner stop and hold machine at the top of each zone)

- Body weight squats-1x6-30-second iso-squats (2 at each of 3 zones)(Have partner hold your shoulders to prevent movement at the top of each zone)

Shoulders 211

- Front lateral raises-1x6-30-second iso-raises (2 at each of 3 zones)(Lift your arms against a machine or wall at the top of each zone)

Triceps

- Static press-downs- 1x6-30-second iso-presses (2 at each of 3 zones)(Have partner hold weight stack to stop movement at the top of each zone)

Biceps

- Chin-ups-1x6-30-second iso-pulls (2 at each of 3 zones)(Have partner hold body to stop movement at the top of each zone)

Forearms

- Grip squeezes-1x6-30-second iso-squeezes (2 at each of 3 zones)(Squeeze hard statically at each zone)

Abs

- Lying leg raises- 1x6-30-second iso-raises (2 at each of 3 zones)(Have partner hold body to stop movement at the top of each zone)

These routines are great to use as an alternative to other HIT routines or as part of a superset. The object of this training is to avoid the lifting of weight and use pure isometric contractions instead. If using as a superset, complete all free weight sets for a muscle group before doing the isometrics.

Full Body HIT Routines #1   212

Chest

- Decline dumbbell flyes- 1x12

- Incline machine bench press-1x8

Back

- Chin-ups- 1x12
- End barbell rows- 1x8
- Stiff-legged deadlift- 1x 8

Legs

- Barbell squat- 1x12
- Leg press- 1x15
- Standing leg curl- 1x12
- Standing calf raises- 1x20

Shoulders

- Front cable raises- 1x12
- Seated machine presses- 1x8

Biceps

- Drag barbell curls- 1x10
- Dumbbell concentration curls- 1x10

Triceps

- Seated machine triceps extensions- 1x12
- Reverse barbell bench presses- 1x8

Abs

- Lying leg raises- 1x25
- Incline sit-ups- 1x25

Forearms

- Grip machine squeezes- 1x15

Full Body HIT Routines #2

Legs

- Leg extensions- 1x20
- Barbell hack squats- 1x12
- Seated calf raises- 1x20

Chest

- Cable crossovers- 1x15
- Flat dumbbell bench press- 1x6

Back

- Seated machine rows-1x8
- High cable rows-1x12
- Machine back extensions-1x12

Shoulders

- Dumbbell shoulder shrugs-1x8
- Incline dumbbell shoulder raise-1x12

Biceps

- Dumbbell concentration curls-1x12
- Machine curls-1x8

Triceps

- Standing cable power push-downs-1x10
- Standing bar dips-1x8

Abs

- Incline sit-ups-1x20

Forearms

- Gripper squeezes-1x25

Pre-exhaust Full Body HIT Routine

Legs

- Leg extensions-1x20
- Hack squat-1x12
- Leg curls-1x15
- Stiff-legged deadlift-1x12
- Toe presses on leg press machine-1x20

Back

- Stiff-arm lat pull-downs-1x12
- End barbell rows-1x8
- Good mornings-1x12
- Deadlifts-1x8

Chest

- Decline dumbbell flyes-1x12
- Flat bench barbell bench press-1x6

Shoulders

- Front dumbbell lateral raise-1x12
- Alternating dumbbell press-1x8

Biceps

- Cable preacher curls-1x12
- Palms-facing pull-ups-1x10

Triceps

- Dumbbell triceps kickbacks-1x12
- Reverse barbell bench press-1x6

Forearms

- Wind-ups-1x4
- Reverse barbell curls-1x8

Abs

- Hanging knee raises-1x25
- Ab wheel-1x12

Split Routines

I have outlined many effective routines for all types of HIT training for each muscle group but, with the exception of full body routines, haven't outlined an appropriate schedule to group them together for efficiency and maximum gains. 216 I discussed frequency of training, which when followed properly, results in relatively quick recuperation, growth and resumption of training at the proper time.

Both frequency of training and proper formation of workouts are imperative to maximize the results obtained from your bodybuilding efforts. If training is repeated too soon before a muscle has had adequate time to recover a bodybuilder won't be able to put forth enough exertion to stimulate a growth response in the muscle. The CNS, or central nervous system will suffer as well and will lead to a feeling of being run down and constantly out of energy.

Not only is it important to avoid training a muscle too often, its equally important to allow the body to recuperate overall. While there are guidelines to use, bodybuilders and trainers must take into consideration the individual bodybuilder's unique recuperative capacity. For instance, bodybuilder A may be able to retrain his/her biceps 7 days after training them previously while bodybuilder B may have to wait 10-12 days.

To come up with the ideal regimen it will take some trial and error. If you train your chest on Monday and all soreness and feeling of depletion in the muscle is gone by the following Monday, try training chest again. If your strength increases a little bit and your energy level is high, then you have determined your ideal frequency. If your strength has decreased and/or you have a diminished energy level, cease training and rest three additional days before trying again.

Split Schedule-2 days   217

Tuesday

- Legs,Back,Abs

Friday

- Chest,Shoulders,Biceps,Triceps, Forearms

Split Schedule-3 days

Monday

- Chest,Back

Wednesday

- Legs,Abs

Friday

Shoulders, Biceps,Triceps

Push-Pull Schedule

Monday

- Chest,Shoulders,Triceps

Wednesday

- Back,Biceps, Abs

Friday

- Legs

Isolation -Compound Exercises

Isolation

Legs

- Leg extensions
- Leg curls
- Dumbbell step-ups

- Leg abductor

- Leg adduction

- Standing calf raises

- Seated calf raises

- Toe presses

Compound Exercises

Legs

- Barbell squat

- Front squat

- Dumbbell squat

- Barbell hack squat

- Machine hack squat

- Leg press

- Dumbbell leg lunges

- Stiff-legged deadlift

- Good mornings

- Reverse hack squat

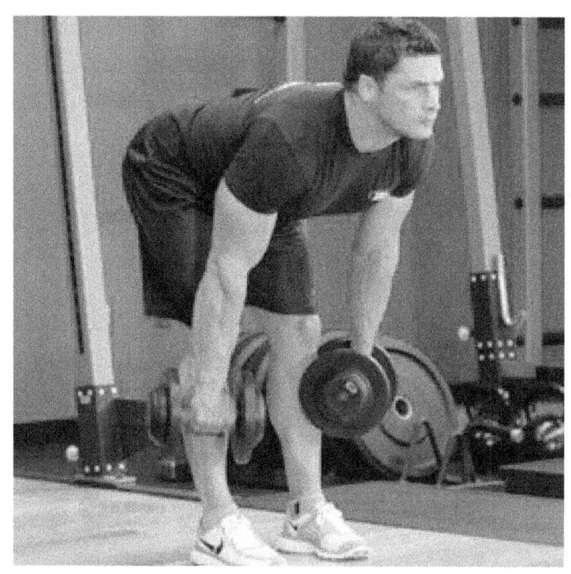

Stiff-legged dead-lift-start

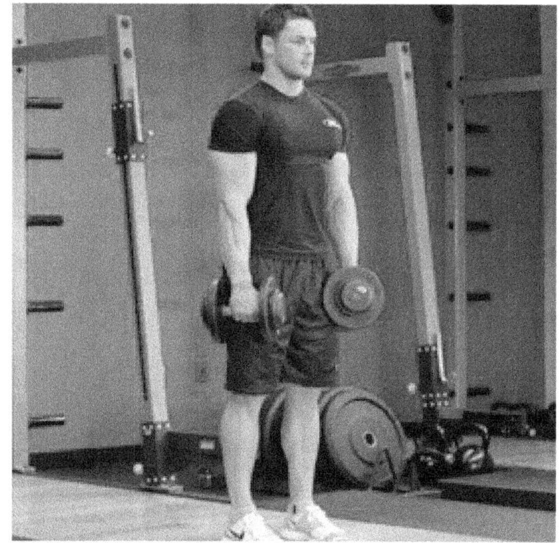

Stiff-legged dead-lift-end

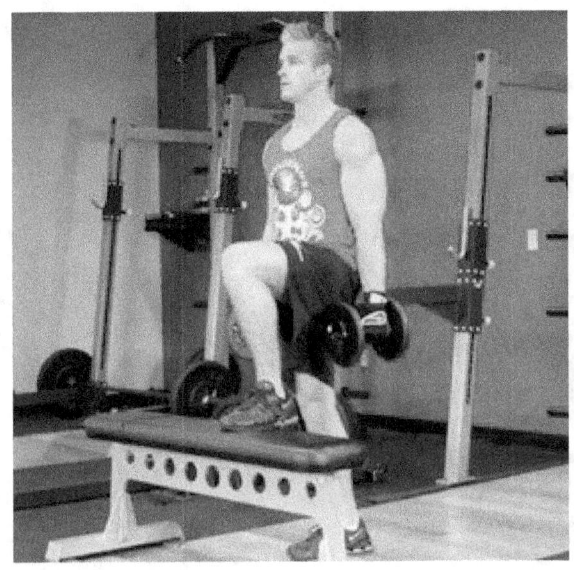

Dumbbell step-ups

Isolation Exercises

Chest

- Pek dek flyes
- Incline dumbbell flyes
- Flat dumbbell flyes
- Decline dumbbell flyes
- High-pulley cable crossovers
- Mid-pulley cable crossovers
- Low-pulley cable crossovers

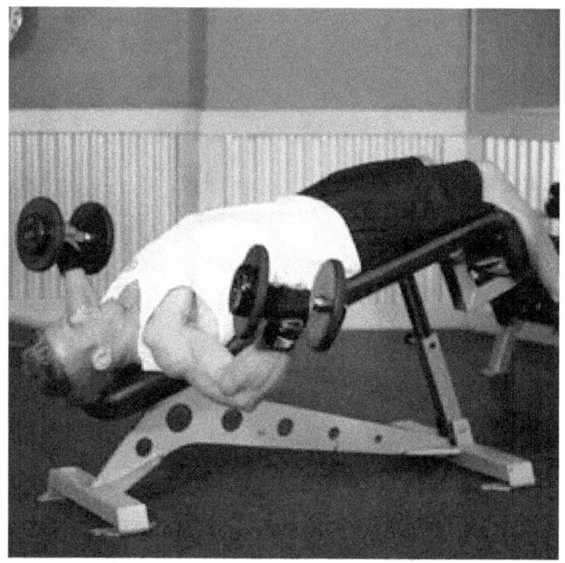

Decline dumbbell flyes

Compound Exercises

Chest

- Barbell bench press
- Barbell incline bench press
- Barbell decline bench press
- Dumbbell incline bench press
- Dumbbell bench press
- Dumbbell decline bench press
- Incline machine bench press
- Machine bench press
- Decline machine bench press
- Standing bar dips

- Machine dips
- Push-ups

Isolation Exercises

Back

- Stiff-arm lat pull-down
- Nautilus pullover
- Dumbbell bench pullover
- Ab strap bent-arm pull-down
- Reverse pek dek flyes

Compound Exercises

Back

- Lat pull-down
- End barbell row
- Barbell row
- Dumbbell row
- One-arm dumbbell row
- Seated machine row
- Chin-up
- Pull-ups
- Seated cable row
- V-handle lat pull-down
- High cable row

- Barbell deadlift

Isolation Exercises

Shoulders

- Seated machine lateral raise
- Standing front lateral raise
- Standing side lateral raise
- Bent-over lateral raise
- Barbell upright row
- Dumbbell upright row
- Cable upright row
- Incline dumbbell side lateral raise
- Incline front lateral raise
- Kettlebell round the worlds(body)
- Dumbbell rotator cuff rotations

Compound Exercises

Shoulders

- Barbell press
- Seated barbell press
- Seated dumbbell press
- Barbell shrugs
- Dumbbell shrugs
- Barbell cleans

Isolation Exercises

Biceps

- Barbell curl
- Dumbbell curl
- Barbell drag curl
- Close-grip barbell curl
- Wide-grip barbell curl
- Dumbbell hammer curl
- Cable hammer curl
- Dumbbell concentration curl
- Barbell preacher curl
- Dumbbell preacher curl
- Cable preacher curl
- Barbell Scott curl
- Dumbbell Scott curl
- Seated rope side curl
- Seated rope overhead curl
- Incline dumbbell curl
- Lying flat dumbbell curl
- Lying incline dumbbell curl
- Cable curl
- Machine curl

- Nautilus overhead machine curl

- Zottman curl

- Bicep Bomber barbell curls

- Cross-body dumbbell hammer curl

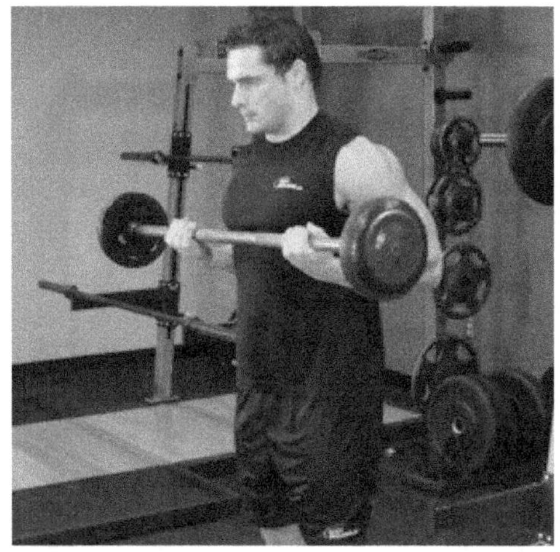

Barbell drag curl

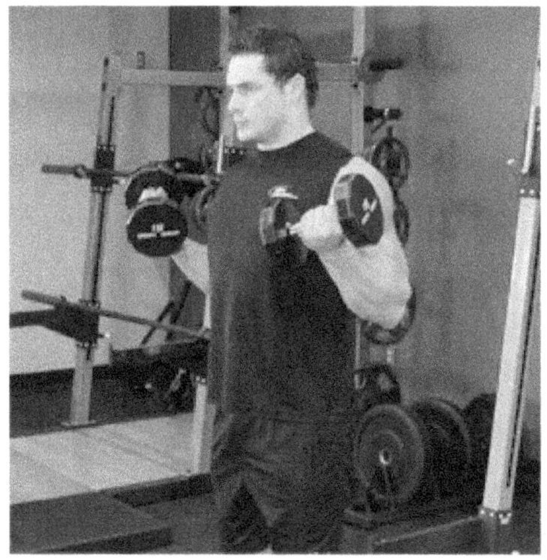

Zottman curl-top

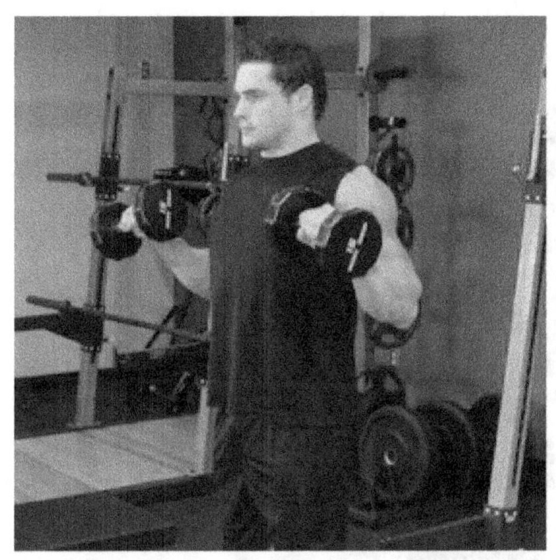

Zottman curl-mid-point

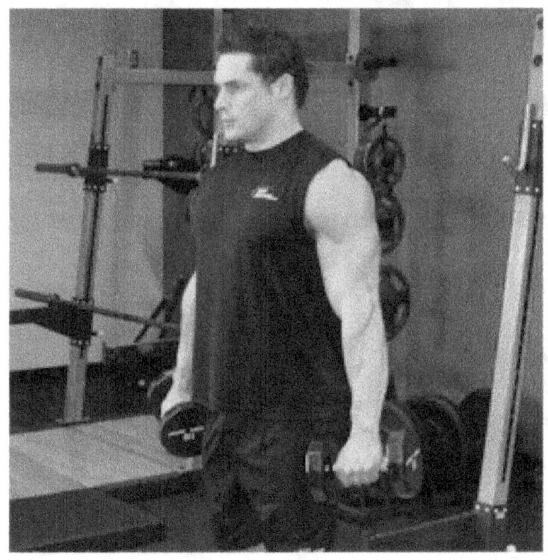

Zottman curl-end

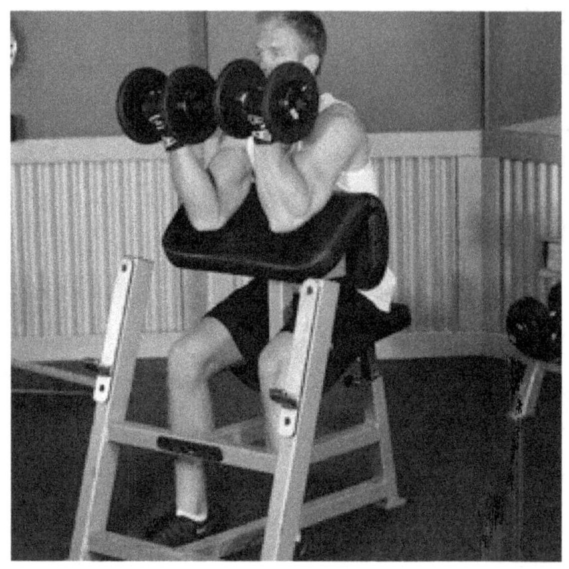

Dumbbell preacher curl

Compound Exercises

Biceps

- Palms-forward barbell row

- Palms-forward machine row

- Palms-facing lat pull-down

- Palms-forward dumbbell row

- Chin-up

- Rope palms-facing overhead row

- Rope mid-pulley palms-up row

Isolation Exercises   228

Triceps

- Standing cable push-down
- Standing cable power push-down
- Standing cable press-down
- Seated high-pulley tricep extension
- Seated mid-pulley tricep extension
- Standing high-pulley tricep extension
- Seated dumbbell overhead tricep extension
- Seated machine tricep extension
- Lying barbell tricep extension
- Dumbbell kickback
- Cable kickback
- Band kickback
- Barbell kickback
- Reverse-grip dumbbell kickback
- Cross-face dumbbell tricep extension
- One-arm cable press-down
- One-arm reverse-grip cable press-down

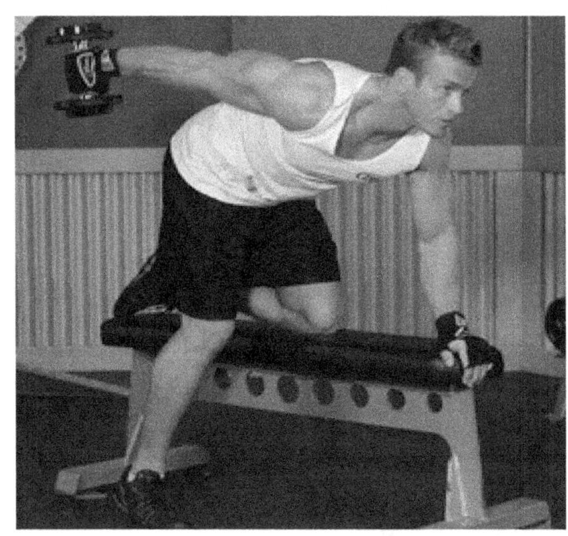

Dumbbell triceps kickback

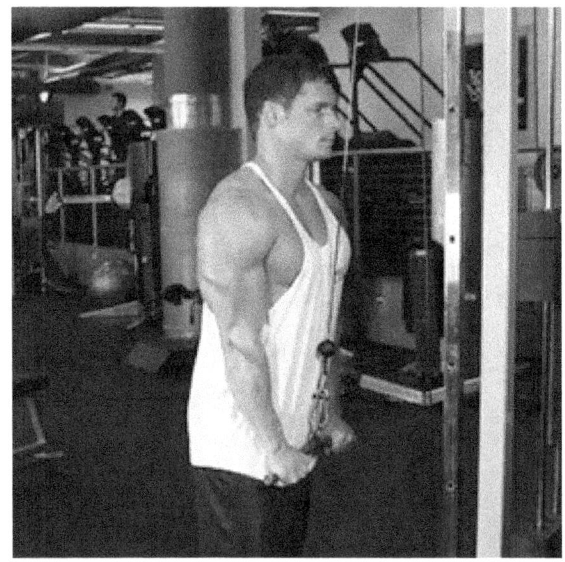

Triceps cable push-downs

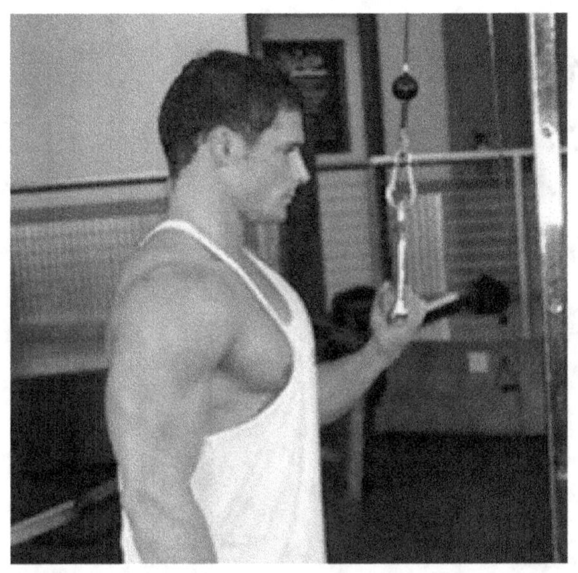

One-arm reverse-grip cable tricep push-down

Compound Exercises

Triceps

- Close-grip barbell bench press
- Close dumbbell neutral-grip bench press
- Reverse-grip barbell bench press
- Standing bar tricep dips
- Seated machine tricep dips
- Bench dips
- Top partial machine bench press
- Close-grip push-up

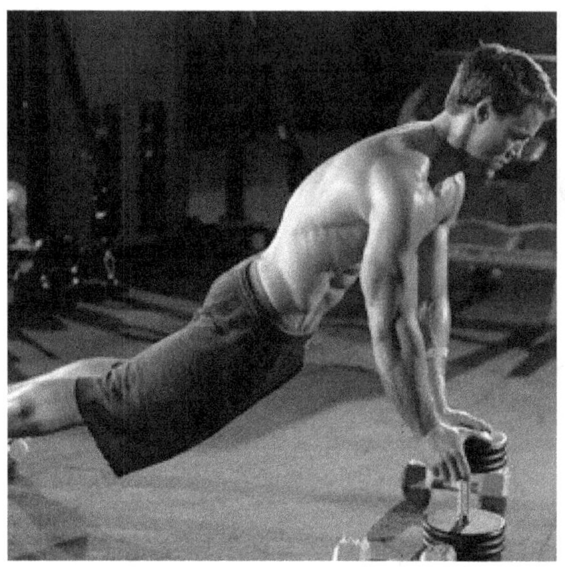

Close-grip push-up off dumbbell

Forearm

Isolation and Compound Exercises

- Barbell wrist curls
- Barbell reverse wrist curls
- Wind-ups
- Gripper squeezes
- Barbell plate pinch grip
- Plate-loaded grip machine
- Grip ball squeezes
- Rotation twists
- Reverse barbell curls

232

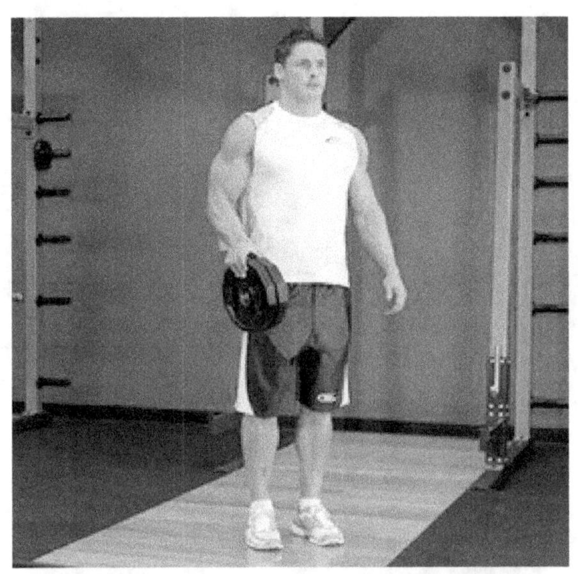

Barbell plate pinch-grip

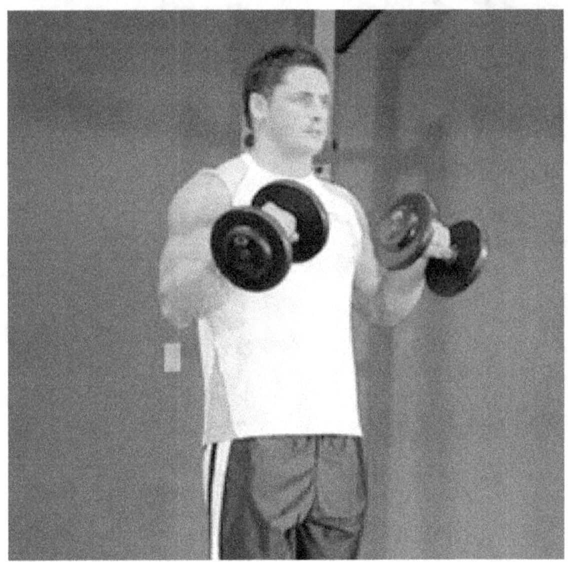

Dumbbell reverse curl

Isolation and Compound Exercises

- Machine crunches
- Machine leg raises
- Hanging leg raises
- Lying leg raises
- Incline bench leg raises
- Sit-ups
- Incline sit-ups
- Ab crunches

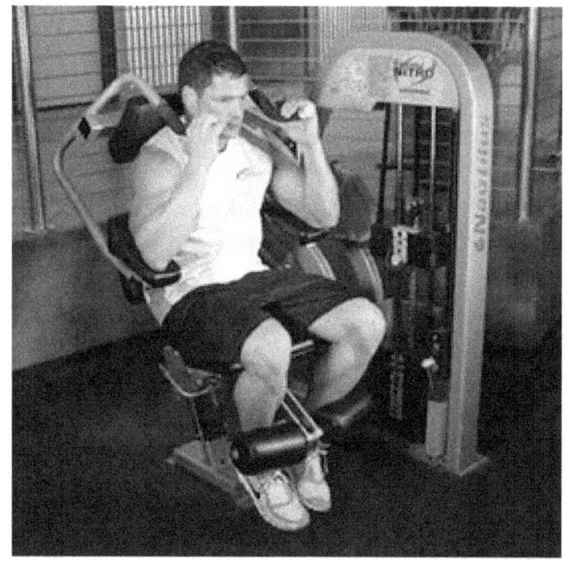

Machine crunches

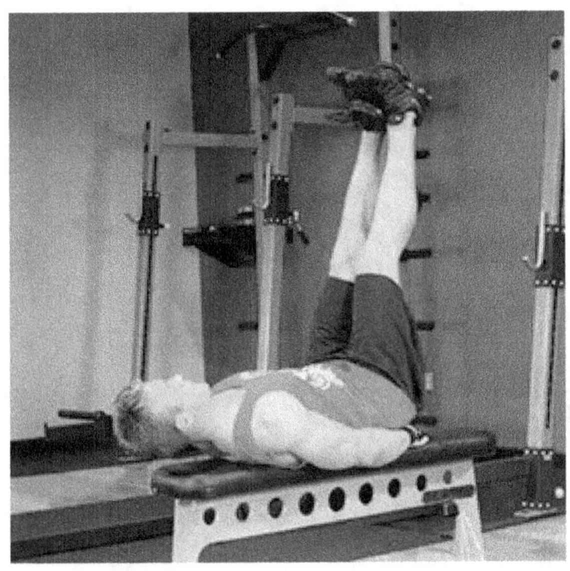

Lying leg raises

Questions and Answers

Q. I have been doing 8 intense sets total for my back training but my gains have stopped for some reason. Should I add some extra sets to help my back to grow?

A. No. This is a very common temptation and springs from the saying "If some is good, more is better." I recommend reducing your sets to a total of three(3) spread out over three exercises (one set of each exercise). Train your back once a week and remain focused on taking each set to total failure by training as hard as you possibly can using the different HIT techniques outlined in this book.

Q. Can I use more than one HIT variable during a single set?

A. Yes. A typical set in HIT is taken to momentary muscular failure, when no more full reps can be completed. To   235 make the set more intense HIT variables are added usually at the end of the set. These consist of forced reps, negative reps and the like. A set using forced reps would look like this: after completing 8 reps and failing to grind out more, your training partner assists with just enough force to allow you to finish 3 additional reps. The set ends at this point.

But a bodybuilder can increase the intensity by adding several negative reps after completing the 3 forced reps. To do this,your partner lifts the bar or machine's arms under his/her strength and transfer the weight to you. You then lower the weight to a count of 8. There are other combinations that can be done as well. Remember to reduce the set count to compensate for the added intensity.

Q. What is progressive overload?

A. Progressive overload is the gradual increase in the demands placed on a muscle. During HIT training, and other systems as well, bodybuilders attempt to gain muscle by overloading their muscles. HIT trainees train with maximum intensity almost always , while medium volume and high volume trainees use a higher volume-less intensity approach.

Both groups attempt to increase the weight used during an exercise in an effort to place greater demands on the muscle and make it grow. This is progressive overload- the adding of a relatively small amount of weight during each workout session. Double-progressive overload is the adding of weight and the increase of rep count in an exercise-something that is very effective at driving both strength and muscle mass.   236

Q. I have used the press-behind neck for delt training and lat pull-downs behind neck for back training but noticed you exclude them from your training routines.

A. They are not a part of my training programs because they can cause major problems with your shoulders due to impingement of your shoulder girdle, most specifically your rotator cuff region. To illustrate this, use a light weight to do a few press-behind neck reps.

As you bring the bar down to your shoulders you will notice that your shoulder is "pinned down" by the weight. This stretches the ligaments in the area and opens you to a risk of shoulder injury. The same occurs during the lat pull-down behind-neck exercise, so please avoid these.

Q. I'm having trouble gaining muscle size even though I work really hard in training. I have had good strength gains. Why no size?

A. Since you didn't mention how long this has been taking place, I'll assume that this has been a fairly recent situation for you. It is very common for a bodybuilder to experience an increase in strength prior to muscle size gains. Many bodybuilders aim to get a good pump during their workouts and aren't overly concerned about strength gains. They are missing the point and need to realize the importance of measuring strength gains as they precede muscle hypertrophy as mentioned above. Train hard and the size gains will come.

Q. Was there a full-body routine used by the Nautilus

group?

A. Arthur Jones, inventor of Nautilus Equipment, advocated a full-body routine to be done three times per week. He promoted this in the 1970's and it was used with good success by HIT bodybuilders Mike and Ray Mentzer and others. Mike later realized that because he was training his entire body during the same workout, he was unable to generate maximum intensity while training muscles later in his workout.

He changed to a split routine in which he trained several muscles together during the first workout and the remaining muscles during the second. This worked much better since his intensity increased dramatically during both sessions since he was fully refreshed at the beginning of each session.

Q. Is there an ideal rep range for developing strength and another for adding muscle size or is it best to do the same rep range for each?

A. While its true that lifting weights with any rep range will develop some strength and size, there are different ideal rep ranges for developing strength and muscle size. To maximize strength gains and limit size gains, use a rep range of 2-5 and rest 3 minutes between sets. The rest period allows the muscles to recuperate enough to be ready for maximum strength output.

Size gains are best realized using moderate weights and reps, in the range of 8-12. To combine strength and muscle size gains use a rep count of 6-10. These recommendations   238 are the result of extensive testing and studies proving them to be effective.

Q. Related to the last question, I have seen powerlifters who aren't large, and in fact barely look like they lift weights, lift enormous poundages during training and powerlifting meets. How can they lift more than lifters who are much larger?

A. There are several reasons for this. Certain lifters have a genetic predisposition for having very efficient neuromuscular efficiency. This means they are able to recruit a much larger number of muscle fibers which enables them to lift heavier weights than others.

Another reason is practice. The more a lifter practices the various lifts, the better he/she gets at executing them. A final reason could be the lifter's training regimen. If trained by an experienced trainer, the lifter bypasses mistakes,trains more efficiently and is more productive in their workouts.

Q. Is there any value in using isometric training to build strength?

A. Yes. While I don't recommend the use of isometrics exclusively to build strength, they are a very useful tool to recruit a high amount of muscle fibers and exert a great amount of stress on a muscle safely if done properly.

Isometrics resemble static holds in which a heavy weight is held motionless for a period of time in the respect that isometrics exert muscular force against an immovable object for a predetermined time under tension. See the section on Isometric Training for specifics on using this valuable   239 tool to increase the effectiveness of your training.

Conclusion

In conclusion, I would like to thank you for purchasing my book and ask that you follow the programs in it faithfully. This will accelerate your gains in muscle size and strength and aid you in developing the physique you desire.

Many different techniques and programs have been offered to Medium-Volume and HIT trainees alike to expand and improve the tools available to help you realize better results from your training. Read through all of my books and visit my blog at: http://drhitshighintensitybodybuilding.blogspot.com/ for more information on bodybuilding training.

Best of luck in bodybuilding,

Dave Groscup

IART/Med-ex HIT Trainer

Certified Nutritional Therapist

Certified Sports Nutritionist

Best-selling author

Over 40 years training experience

www.ingramcontent.com/pod-product-compliance
Lightning Source LLC
Chambersburg PA
CBHW080900160726
48000CB00009B/2795